the nervous girl's guide to
nip & tuck

Look 10 years younger
with **80 no-surgery** treatments

Dr Patrick Bowler

with Jennifer Christie

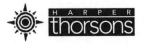

HARPER
thorsons

To my wife Pauline and my family,
without whom I could not do what I do!

HarperThorsons
An Imprint of HarperCollins*Publishers*
77–85 Fulham Palace Road,
Hammersmith, London W6 8JB

The website address is: www.thorsonselement.com

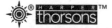

and *HarperThorsons* are trademarks of
HarperCollins*Publishers* Ltd

First published by HarperThorsons 2006

10 9 8 7 6 5 4 2 1

© 2006 Patrick Bowler

Patrick Bowler asserts the moral right to be
identified as the author of this work

Botox®, Retin-A®, Dianette®, Yasmin®, Roaccutane® and Vistabel® are all registered trademarks.
References in this book to trademarks and prescription medicines are for clarification only.

A catalogue record of this book is
available from the British Library

ISBN-13 978-0-00-722548-4
ISBN-10 0-00-722548-2

Printed and bound in Great Britain by
Clays Ltd, St Ives plc

Contents

No-Surgery Treatments for Lips 45

No-Surgery Treatments for Cheeks 57

No-Surgery Treatments for the Trunk, Front and Back 135

No-Surgery Treatments for Legs 145

No-Surgery Treatments for Anywhere 157

Part two

The aim of this book is to inform you about treatments currently available, how they work and what to expect, without boring you with medical jargon.

I have arranged Part One so that each area of the face and body is covered by a separate chapter, to make it easy for you to locate any personal issues you have and find out which no-surgery techniques we use to treat them. I have included the most common cosmetic issues my patients experience and left out obscure ones that are unlikely to be relevant to most readers. Sometimes, if a problem could crop up in one or two different areas of the face or body, I have included it under the area where it bothers people most, so if you can't find what you're looking for, check the index and see if it's covered elsewhere.

Should you want to find out more about a particular no-surgery technique you've heard of or read about in Part One, turn to Part Two for more details. Also included in Part Two are first-hand accounts from some of my patients, describing what the treatments felt like and what results they had, to give you a different perspective.

I also felt it was important to mention common cosmetic problems for which there are, as yet, no effective treatments – not to disappoint you but to measure your expectations and deter you from wasting your money on treatments that won't give you a good result. Don't be discouraged. In the final chapter of Part Two you can read about exciting new no-surgery techniques being developed to enable cosmetic doctors and specialists to treat these stubborn problems in future. Some of these new treatments are due to be launched in the next couple of years.

Whether this is your first step towards trying no-surgery treatments or you have already tried them but want to know more, I hope this book helps you find an experienced practitioner and enjoy a good result.

Dr Patrick Bowler

Introduction

> *'I'm very nervous. I don't know why, Doctor,*
> *but I am very nervous.'*

Nervous is a good description of the people who usually
come to see me. Most people come via a very circuitous
route. They've read something in a magazine or heard it
through a friend and think carefully before they make 'that
phone call'. They are often sceptical and embarrassed. So the
first thing I always do is try to put them at ease and answer
all their questions. You have to gain their confidence. This is
an important and interesting part of my job.

Sometimes I get visitors whose problems are more
psychological than physical – once a month on average.
These patients have a serious condition known as body
dysmorphic disorder. In general they are young and have
beautiful features but they believe they are ugly. One of the
first clues is that they come in with their own magnifying
mirror and look into it while repeating idealistic
expressions like 'disappear' and 'perfect'. This condition is
like anorexia in that these patients have a false body image.
They become obsessed with disfiguring scars, wrinkles and
blemishes that are barely noticeable. In America, forty per
cent of people who go to see a cosmetic surgeon have some
degree of body dysmorphism.

A mother once came in to see me with her 18-year-old
daughter. The girl was unhappy about a scar on her cheek.
I couldn't see anything. I had some new glasses and thought

this could be the problem, so I got out my magnifying glass and after another good look I said, 'I'm sorry, I can't really see what's bothering you.' This made the girl very upset and she had a good shout at me before storming off, leaving her mother in the room. Her mother just got up and thanked me. 'She won't leave the house,' she said. 'We've been telling her there's nothing there but she won't believe us.'

The sad thing is that people like this will go somewhere else and, eventually, someone might take advantage of them and treat them when it's not necessary. What they really need is a psychological approach to help them resolve their problem.

However, the majority of my first-time patients have a balanced perspective. They want a few inhibiting cosmetic problems sorted out, so they can feel themselves again and get on with their lives. The self-improvement movement has spawned dozens of TV programmes dedicated to making-over faces, bodies and wardrobes, all of which demonstrate the positive impact this has on people's confidence.

The number of visitors to my clinics has doubled each year for the last five years, and other cosmetic doctors I chat to say they are just as busy. Two to three times a week journalists call me with questions about cosmetic treatments. Every day I have questions from the public through my clinic website. Once, immediately after I had appeared on a TV programme, I was asked to host a web chat. Viewers emailed their questions and at one point I remember there were over 300 waiting. An hour later there was still a queue. Eventually, we had to call a halt and the questions were diverted to my website. I spent the following week trying to catch up! I was genuinely surprised by the response, and impressed by the type of questions being asked. There is clearly a demand for information on non-surgical treatments. So I've decided to pen you this guide.

Questions answered

☆ What is available?

☆ What can they do?

☆ How much should I expect to pay?

☆ How do they work?

☆ How well do they work?

☆ Which don't work?

☆ Will it hurt?

☆ Are there any risks or side-effects?

☆ When will I see the results?

☆ How long will the results last?

Although you can get such information from the internet there is a lot of sales rubbish on it too. So how do you know which bits are true? After all, people can put anything they like on there. Every month a new treatment comes on to the marketplace, some good, some useless, some downright dangerous. However, you can be sure that I am only interested in telling you the truth – my career depends on it!

I also have a personal motive for writing this book. It provides me with an opportunity to emphasize the importance of seeking no-surgery treatments from a medically qualified cosmetic doctor. At the time of writing it is still possible for consumers in the UK to go to a beauty salon and have botox injections given by a beautician – sometimes with disastrous results. This book will arm you with information on how to avoid a bad result, so you can safely and assuredly reap the benefits that no-surgery treatments can offer.

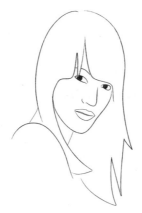

A bit about me

I just had to write and thank you once again for helping to turn me into a very pretty lady. The difference is amazing and I am so happy with the end results. My skin feels really lovely and now I have the knowledge of how to look after it. As for my lips, they look stunning. Must go now as I have been away from the mirror for at least 15 mins and I'm getting withdrawal symptoms!

This was the letter I had from Bernie Sharp, the first lady we treated on the TV series '10 Years Younger in 10 Days'. Wouldn't you feel rewarded if you got a letter like this?

My mission is to make someone look as good as they can – not necessarily as young as they can, but as good as they can. This usually takes a combination of treatments: smoothing out lines, removing any lumps and bumps, as well as skin-improvement treatments and some decent skincare they can use at home. I want people to understand that it is not just a bit of botox – that we have more to offer. Someone might walk into the clinic and say, 'I've got this permanently frowning expression. Can you give me some botox?' A good cosmetic doctor worth their salt can do much more – they can do a lot of little things to get an overall improvement.

My patients

The problems are very personal. When people walk into my clinic, I can't help trying to guess what they are going to tell me. One lady who came in to see me had an enormous mole on her top lip. It was the sort of thing your eyes are magnetically attracted to. Of course, it wasn't what she came in for: she was bothered by a small scar on the side of her face. I helped her sort that out. Then, once I had got to know her better and gained her confidence, I plucked up a bit of courage and said, 'What about that mole on your top lip?' She said, 'What mole?'

I've learned it is better to start by asking rather than suggesting. Obviously, the mole wasn't an issue for her. You have to get to know someone well and gain their trust first, then sometimes, if it is appropriate, you can make suggestions. This patient came back at a later date and we ended up removing the mole.

What are 'no-surgery' treatments?

We are on a new wave of exciting changes in no-surgery procedures in the UK.

When I first started doing this in 1987, collagen injections, sclerotherapy and peels were the only clinical aesthetic treatments available that didn't involve major surgery. Now there are a range of treatments like these, which share four defining characteristics:

1. They can physically alter your skin without damaging it

No-surgery treatments work by changing the structure of the skin without leaving it damaged, and the benefits are long-lasting: from six months to a year, and in some cases beyond. Sometimes no-surgery treatments offer permanent solutions to problems even surgery can't resolve.

2. They don't stop your life

No-surgery treatments are relatively painless. None of these treatments needs a general anaesthetic or a stay in hospital.

The treatment sessions are short – most take less than 15 minutes – and they don't involve any downtime so you can walk out and get on with your life.

3. They are discreet

We're talking subtle improvements. No-surgery treatments offer a more discreet way to improve our looks than surgery does – a tweak here and there or a change that develops gradually with a series of treatments. Nobody needs to know you've had anything done. Provided you go to an experienced practitioner, the improvements are generally very subtle. After treatment, the reaction my patients get from friends and loved ones is that they look 'great' or 'radiant' – which is exactly the result that they wanted.

4. They cost less than surgery

Surgery is expensive because of all the razzmatazz – consultants, anaesthetists, hospital beds, drugs – so there are big savings to be made when it is less than an hour spent with just one specialist.

Where do you get them?

1. Cosmetic doctors

In the mid-nineties, doctors working in the NHS began supplementing their income with a bit of outside work. Eye surgeons, GPs, ear, nose and throat specialists and dermatologists started practising 'aesthetic treatments', which I refer to in this book as 'no-surgery treatments' to clearly distinguish them from cosmetic surgery.

Cosmetic doctors grew as the number of no-surgery treatments expanded and doctors moved across to specialize in them. To help the public understand the difference between plastic surgeons and cosmetic doctors I co-founded the Cosmetic Doctors Association with 25 doctor members. We now have 200 in Great Britain and Ireland, all specializing in no-surgery techniques. Our members meet regularly and attend training courses to keep them up to date on new techniques.

2. Aesthetic nurses

Nurses specifically trained in cosmetic work can give you any no-surgery treatments. Those that require a prescription, like botox and microsclerotherapy, must be done under a doctor's supervision. By this I mean the doctor must assess and examine you, prescribe the treatment and then remain near enough to be on hand while the nurse is treating you.

3. Beauty therapists

Beauty therapists can perform some no-surgery treatments, such as light rejuvenation and hair removal, but others, such as botox and sclerotherapy, have to be administered by a cosmetic doctor, because these products are classified as drugs.

4. Dermatologists

There is a shortage of dermatologists in the UK and their time is taken up with work on skin diseases. A few do cosmetic treatments in the UK but there are far more dermatologists offering them in the US.

5. GPs

A few minor surgical procedures can be carried out in your local practice if they are deemed to be medical problems rather than purely cosmetic ones.

6. *Surgeons*

Plastic surgeons deal with birthmarks, burns, injuries
and repairs. They don't get NHS training in no-surgery
techniques, other than laser treatments. If a surgeon does
offer you no-surgery treatments, ask them where they
trained in these procedures before you allow them to
practise them on you. Plastic surgeons do not get NHS
training in cosmetic surgery either. They used to, but the
government stopped this when the NHS ended up paying
for too many nose jobs and breast enhancements on the
grounds that patients were psychologically affected by their
condition. Qualified plastic surgeons wanting to become
cosmetic surgeons have to get themselves trained, usually
by going abroad.

Part 1

No-surgery treatments by area

- ☆ which ones work and which don't
- ☆ how much they will cost
- ☆ how long they will take
- ☆ how long the effects will last
- ☆ how much they will hurt
- ☆ tips, tricks and advice

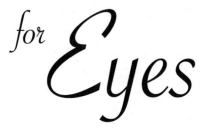

No-Surgery Treatments for Eyes

Psychologists tell us that when we meet someone for the first time we zone in on the 'triangle' formed by their eyes and mouth to decide how attractive they are. It's all to do with the mating instinct. Our eyes form two corners of this triangle, so the more obvious they are, the more attractive we are deemed to be. It's a cruel irony then, isn't it, that the area around our eyes is one of the first to give the game away when it comes to ageing. So why does this happen?

The skin around our eyes is much thinner than the skin on other parts of our face and there is less chubby fat supporting it (try gently pinching the skin under your eye and then do the same on your cheek and you'll feel the difference in thickness). Because it's so thin, it is the first part of our face to lose its stretchiness, and when it does those smiling/squinting lines stop pinging back and become permanent fixtures.

We can blame the weather too. This delicate skin sits on top of our cheekbones – semicircles perfectly positioned to catch the maximum number of UV rays.

Some see age-related changes around their eyes in their late thirties, while others notice them as young as in their late twenties. But even at this age there is a lot we can do with no-surgery treatments to turn back the clock and slow down the rate of further damage, especially if you combine these treatments with a few good habits.

Things that affect how fast we age

Factors in ageing	Who/what to blame
Skin type	Parents
Amount of sun	Weather
Whether we smoke	Stress levels
Stress levels	Boss/boyfriend/parents
Skin care routine	Ourselves
What we eat/drink	All of the above

Common problems

☆ wrinkles

☆ bags

☆ droopy top lids

☆ dark circles

My patients usually have an issue with one or more of these main categories. Not all of these will necessarily be problems for you, of course. A lot depends on your skin type and family history. In the next section I take each one of these categories in turn and explain which no-surgery treatments can be used to treat them. I also suggest any effective action you can take yourself.

Wrinkles around the eyes

Over time our laughter lines – those little branching wrinkles at the outer corners of our eyes that appear when we smile or squint – become permanent and earn the less endearing title of 'crow's feet'. The severity of your crow's feet depends a lot on your lifestyle. Spend a lot of time outdoors where it is bright and you are bound to squint more. If you are looking after customers you will need to smile more. The more you work the muscles the stronger they will get; and the stronger the muscles are, the more forcefully they deepen the lines. I also suspect heavy-handedly applying eye makeup or removing contact lenses can contribute to these wrinkles – if you are repeatedly rough with this area you can overstretch the skin, making it lose its elasticity sooner than it would have otherwise.

These expression lines should be differentiated from the much finer lines which form just underneath our eyes. When and where we get these finer lines depends on our genes and how much sun we've had.

What you can do

☆ I know, I know – you've heard it hundreds of times before, but good skincare habits do make a big difference. There is no point investing in no-surgery treatments unless you are going to look after your new complexion. So discover your inner

20

celeb: wear shades whenever possible, and wear a makeup or moisturizer with a 'built-in' sun barrier – not just when it is sunny but from March through to October. Even the dismal British weather isn't enough to deter the resolute UVA ray.

☆ Respect the fragility of the area around the eyes. Repeatedly stretching and rubbing this delicate skin will make it lose its elasticity sooner: don't rub too much when you remove makeup and be gentle when you are putting it on.

☆ Moisturize the area with creams that contain glycolic acid, vitamin A, vitamin C and Idebenone. Studies have shown that these ingredients all help your skin regenerate itself.

UVA and UVB

Remember 'A' is for ageing and you will remember that UVA rays are the ones mostly responsible for your lines and wrinkles. They travel through clouds and windows and they are there all the time, not just when it is sunny. Remember 'B' for burning and you will remember UVB rays are the ones that give you sunburn. B rays can also cause skin cancer and make your skin age prematurely. The SPF factor on sunscreens only refers to UVB protection. There is no recognized grading system for UVA rays. Just look for the words 'UVA protection' on the label.

Tip

☆ Don't buy a separate product for your eyes – 'eye creams' are a
marketing gimmick. Just use a small amount of the same
cream that you bought for your face instead. Most eye creams
are just milder-strength versions of the face cream, apart from
those that contain a bit of starch (check the ingredients),
which stops the cream spreading onto the eye rim.

Eye bags and puffiness

You'll be relieved to hear that the telltale puffiness you
get under your eyes after a late night or a good cry is only
temporary – it is just a build-up of fluid which drains away
during the course of the day. The 'puffs' that bother my
patients occur when, over time, the natural fatty padding
under their eyes moves down and collects in a ridge shape.
These eye bags, alas, do not disappear by themselves.
What upsets people most is the way their eyes look when
they get that temporary puffiness on top of their bags.
Bags + puffiness = much more obvious puffy bags.

☆ *Tip*

☆ Icepacks, cucumber slices, creams and gels all hasten the
disappearance of the puffiness formed by crying and tiredness.
But watch out where you put the creams and gels. Apply them

too near the lower eyelid and they will seep into the rim, blocking the little ducts that get rid of toxins. If this happens you will end up with double-decker puffs. Keep them roughly half a centimetre beneath the lower lashes and you will be fine. As yet there are no effective home remedies in existence for the bags that develop with age.

Eye bags can be surgically removed. The operation is called a lower blepharoplasty. It is a day case and you would need to consult a surgeon.

Dark circles

Dark circles are a common bugbear apt to appear on anyone, but what makes them more obvious on some than others is still a mystery. When they develop in the teens and twenties it is usually an inherited characteristic. When they appear from the late thirties onwards it is usually age-related.

Two things make the skin here look darker. Firstly, blood vessels and pigment gather in the semi-circular groove beneath the eye, and this gets more obvious over the years as the skin covering it gets thinner. Secondly, loose skin or fat moves downwards over time and gathers in a semicircular ridge, which casts a shadow, making the dark circles look worse.

Cosmetic doctors are busy trying to solve the mystery of dark circles – so far without joy. Attempts to seal the blood vessels using lasers, or erase the pigment using tattoo-removing lasers, haven't worked. Similar to dark circles is the patchy pigmentation around the eyes that typically arises on darker skins, for which again there is as yet no cosmetic solution.

Fillers can be used to plump up the shadowy groove, but we are talking about a very minor improvement. A surgeon can tighten the skin under the eyes to flatten out the semi-circular groove as part of blepharoplasty. It can reduce the shadowing but not the pigmentation.

☆ Tips

☆ Don't buy face creams that claim to treat dark circles – they are a waste of money.

☆ Camouflage dark circles with a concealer that contains the minerals titanium dioxide or zinc dioxide, or both. These minerals are light-reflecting so they do more to lighten the area than just provide a layer of colour.

☆ Opt for a liquid or ground mineral concealer rather than a waxy one (wax concealers are better for blemishes) because they cling to your skin for longer. Wax concealers warm up on the skin and start moving around so they rub off easily.

☆ Keep it subtle: don't sweep concealer under the whole eye, just put it in the hollow close to the inner corner where the dark circle is worst, and blend it outwards into a triangle shape.

Other things that cause a nuisance

Although ageing is responsible for most of our eye-related beauty niggles, no-surgery treatments can also treat other skin conditions that are not necessarily age-related:

☆ spider veins
☆ solar keratosis
☆ fat deposits
☆ syringomas
☆ skin tags
☆ uneven pigmentation

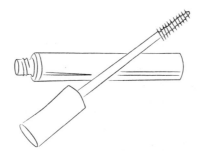

The treatments

I sense you nervous girls becoming a little more nervous at this point. So, let me reassure you. Everything I suggest here is safe, effective and relatively pain-free. And if you are worried about what these no-surgery treatments feel like, you can flick forward to Part Two for full details and first-hand accounts from some of my patients.

I believe that botox and fillers are currently the most effective no-surgery treatments for fine lines, wrinkles and crow's feet, so let's start with these.

Botox for crow's feet

Using botox to relax the smiling/squinting muscles around
the outer corners of the eyes helps prevent you from
developing crow's feet. Not only does it prevent new crow's
feet, but it also reduces any that have already started to show:
you stop reinforcing them, so they gradually fade. And you can
opt for a natural look by using smaller quantities of botox or
selecting to freeze some rather than all of your muscles.

 Tips

☆ If you are going for your first botox treatment, ask the doctor
   to give you the minimum amount you require and then a top-
   up a month later if you need it. I always offer my patients a
   complimentary top-up after their first visit because the
   amount of botox required varies between patients. All good
   practitioners should do this for you.

☆ Botox doesn't always work on the shallower, finer lines that
   gather in the crescent shape just under the eye. It can reduce
   them if the skin there is still fairly elastic, but not if it is loose.
   If it is loose then it is best to look at other options.

Cost: Expect to pay £250–£300 per session.
Patient pain rating: 2–3 (1–10, 1 = pain-free)
Treatment time: 10 minutes
How long does it last? 3–4 months

Microdermabrasion for fine lines

Microdermabrasion removes dead skin cells, which stimulates the growth of new elastic fibres and collagen. As it deeply exfoliates and plumps up the skin, the plumper skin has a more stretched-out surface and therefore looks less wrinkled.

The effect of microdermabrasion on wrinkles is more superficial than botox, but then it doesn't just target individual wrinkles; it improves your complexion by making your skin look smoother. To see an improvement you'll need to have one session a month for six months. After that, you can just have maintenance sessions every three months or so.

☆ *Tips*

☆ This is not suitable for dark skin because occasionally it produces patchy increased pigmentation on darker skin types.

☆ If you have sensitive skin it can make you a little red and sore at first, but it doesn't cause any long-term damage.

☆ Make sure you use a sunscreen for a couple of days after treatment because microdermabrasion removes some of the skin's natural sun protection.

☆ If you don't mind needles, combine microdermabrasion with botox and fillers and you'll really see a difference: the botox and fillers tighten the skin and reduce the wrinkles, while the microdermabrasion plumps the skin up and makes it more radiant.

Cost: Expect to pay £75– £90 for a full face.

Patient pain rating: 2–3 (1–10, 1 = pain-free)

Treatment time: 30 minutes per session

How long does it last? Effects last 2–3 weeks at first, but there is also a cumulative improvement. After an initial course of 6 monthly treatments you should maintain the effects with booster sessions every 2–3 months.

Filling in fine lines

Fillers literally fill in the line – they are the Polyfilla of no-surgery treatments. The filler is injected just underneath the wrinkle, lifting it to make it level with the surrounding skin. Before I start this treatment I like to check how well it will work by performing a quick test. I gently stretch out the wrinkle using my finger and thumb. If, when I do this, the wrinkle disappears, I know that the filler will work well. If the wrinkle does not disappear, I know that using filler will only reduce this wrinkle rather than make it disappear. So remember – your cosmetic doctor should be able to perform this trick for you and tell you what to expect before you decide whether to go ahead.

Cost: Expect to pay £350 per session.
Patient pain rating : 3–4 (1–10, 1 = pain-free) with an anaesthetic
Treatment time: 15 minutes
How long does it last? 6–9 months

Needles? No way. Never!

If you suffer from a condition thought to occur amongst girls of a nervous disposition, known to some as Chronic Needle Phobia, you can opt for no-surgery treatments that plump up the skin to make wrinkles less noticeable.

Intense Pulsed Light (IPL) for fine lines

This is another no-needle treatment that stimulates collagen growth. As with microdermabrasion, the extra collagen plumps up the supporting under-layers, tightening the surface to reduce wrinkles. IPL works better on fairer skins than darker skins. Although it only makes a small difference to wrinkles, compared to the difference you get with botox and fillers, it is good for improving the overall finish of your skin and evening out skin tone.

☆ *Tip*

☆ If you have dark skin, go for a gentle laser instead of IPL, as you are more likely to have side-effects with IPL.

Cost: Expect to pay £250–£300 per session.
Patient pain rating: 5 (1–10, 1 = pain-free)
Treatment time: 5–30 minutes per session
How long does it last? Initial effects last 2–3 months but there is also a cumulative improvement that is long-lasting.

Gentle peels for fine lines

Peeling off the top layers of the skin encourages the lower layers to make more collagen and elastic fibres. It is a different method of achieving the same effect as microdermabrasion and IPL.

Cost: Expect to pay £50 per peel.

Patient pain rating: 1 (1–10, 1 = pain-free)

Treatment time: 30 minutes

How long does it last? 2–3 weeks initially. To build up a long-lasting effect you'll need a course of 5–6 peels a month apart.

Infrared light for fine lines

Red light is a relatively new treatment. We know it is safe, and good clinical studies show it works, but nobody can explain how it works. It is a popular treatment because it is painless and doesn't damage your skin, so there is no recovery time. I've tried it and I think it feels quite pleasant.

The initial plumping, tightening effect is obvious – some of this disappears after the first three days but the rest of it stays there. As with most of these skin-plumping treatments you gradually build up a long-lasting effect by having regular sessions.

☆ *Tip*

☆ Infrared light treatment is a new advance on red light. It works in the same way but it is marginally more effective.

Cost: Expect to pay £75 per session or cheaper for a course.
Patient pain rating: 1 (1–10, 1 = pain-free)
Treatment time: 30 minutes
How long does it last? 2–3 weeks initially. To build up a long-lasting effect you need a course of 5–6 treatments 2–3 months apart.

Laser resurfacing

This is the opposite of the gradual build-up approach. It is the last resort, and it is not a lunchtime procedure. It is considerably more expensive than botox, but it doesn't just reduce wrinkles, it restores your glow. The top layer of skin is removed with a strong laser, wrinkles and all, which in turn triggers the growth of a fresh new layer.

Does it hurt? Well ... yes, so you will need a local anaesthetic (cream or injection), but it is not the treatment itself that is painful, it is the soreness that follows during the recovery time. Resurfacing makes your skin feel and look very raw for two to three weeks, then it stays red for up to six months, and you will have to stay away from the sun for three months. So why do people go through all this? Patients of mine who have had it done say it is painful and inconvenient but the improvement is so dramatic that it is worth it. So, I wouldn't recommend it for anxious types. It is more suitable for severe wrinkles and braver girls.

The same effect can be achieved with strong chemical peels, but I tend to avoid these because peels are less controllable. With a laser you remove the skin little layer by little layer. I feel I can be more accurate this way, which is particularly important when it comes to that delicate thin skin around the eyes.

☆ *Tip*

☆ Enjoy the benefits of laser resurfacing for longer by opting
   for a bit of botox to prevent new wrinkles forming.

Cost: Expect to pay around £1,300 per session (including aftercare
creams and pills to stop infections).

Patient pain rating: 7–8 (1–10, 1 = pain-free)

Treatment time: 30–60 minutes per session

How long does it last? Effects last 3–5 years, or more if you look
after your skin. However, this is a one-off treatment – it is not safe
to repeat it.

Botox brow-lift

The pull of gravity and the stretching effect of facial expressions eventually take their toll on everyone's eyelids and eyebrows, but this happens sooner if your eyebrows and lids are naturally low-set to start with.

This treatment works best on those whose facial muscles are well toned. Two sets of muscles work our brow movements. As you sit attentively making all the right facial expressions while your friend recounts her wild night out, these two sets of muscles are busily conducting a tug of war: one set pulls up and the other set pulls down. Using botox I can relax the muscles that pull down, thereby giving the up-pulling muscles the advantage. So the up-pulling muscles triumph and you get your brow-lift.

While the botox brow-lift pulls up the brow it makes little difference to the lid. You can see what I mean by putting a finger on your forehead and pushing it upwards – it is your brow that moves most, not your lid (at present, no-surgery options are not available for eyelids). How good the results are depends on your muscle tone. Your doctor should be able to give you an idea as to how well it will work on you.

Tip

☆ Ignore lotions, potions or electrical treatments promising to firm up drooping eyelids – they are a waste of money.

☆ People are always surprised when I tell them about this treatment because of the press stories about botox causing droopy eyelids. The only way you can get droopy lids from botox injections is if your doctor gives you too much or puts it in the wrong place – blame the workman, not his tools.

Cost: Expect to pay around £250 per session.
Patient pain rating: 2 (1–10, 1=pain-free)
Treatment time: 10 minutes
How long does it last? 3–5 months

Radiofrequency remodelling

This is an exciting new treatment. Radio waves actually tighten the skin. If you do this between the top lid and eyebrow it even lifts the eyelid a bit. If you have this underneath your eye it tightens the loose crêpey skin a little. The effects continue to improve during the weeks after you have had radio frequency treatment. I've tried it myself and I would describe it as a dull hot sensation.

The technology varies. Some systems require sedation and anaesthetic but others just give you a deep feeling of heat like a burning inside. You get recovery time in between any bouts of discomfort because the pain goes as soon as you lift the probe off. It is more painful around the eyes, forehead and jaw line, where there is bone immediately underneath. It is less painful wherever there is more fat to absorb the heat.

Cost: This will change and vary from doctor to doctor, depending on the type of machine they have. There is a big variation, anything from £500 to £3,500 per session, and you may need 3–4 sessions four weeks apart.

Patient pain rating: 5–6 (1–10, 1 = pain-free) although it varies between machines and different parts of the face.

Treatment time: 45 minutes

How long does it last? 1–2 years as we understand at the moment.

IPL or lasers for spider veins

Spider veins are caused by a single blood vessel rising to the skin's surface and bursting into a visible network of tiny capillaries. They most commonly emerge on the cheekbone and nose, but my patients seem to be more irritated if they get one under their eyes. Protecting your skin from harsh weather will help to prevent them.

Who gets spider veins? Anyone can. Some are born with them, some develop them because they spend long periods exposed to the elements (both the sun and the wind can spark off spider veins). Women often get them during pregnancy and anyone can get them when they are scratched or grazed; my son developed one after a fight with his brother.

Although spider veins sometimes disappear by themselves, they are easy to remove with a laser or IPL. I used a laser to treat my son's spider vein; he described the sensation as a bit like being 'pinged' with an elastic band. It usually takes one or two sessions to get rid of them completely. They can come back, but they are less likely to if you don't overdo it in the sun.

Cost: £100–£200 depending on how many you have.
Patient pain rating: 2–3 (1–10, 1=pain-free)
Treatment time: 5 minutes per session
How long does it last? Effects last forever.

Lasers for solar keratosis

These small, red, raised patches of rough scaly skin congregate round the eyes, temples or forehead. We get them in our sixties and beyond, if we have spent too much time in the sun.

Advice: There is a tiny chance that SK is pre-cancerous so get it checked by your GP. If you are diagnosed with SK wear sunscreens and a hat; further sunning could make it turn cancerous.

Provided they are non-cancerous, SK patches can either be removed layer by layer using a laser, or frozen off using liquid nitrogen. Both treatments hurt a bit, but they work.

☆ *Tip*

☆ I also recommend applying a cancer-treating cream every day for about a month, which prevents them growing any bigger. These creams do have a side-effect – they make the skin blister – but they work. If you keep applying the cream they will eventually scab over and fall off. Discuss this with your GP or dermatologist.

Cost: Expect to pay around £200 per session.
Patient pain rating: 5–6 (1–10, 1=pain-free)
Treatment time: 15–30 minutes per session
How long does it last? The SK disappears but may form again.

Lasers for yellow fatty lumps

Xanthelasma is rare but unsightly. These yellow streaks of fat that crop up near the corner of the eyes can be a sign you have high cholesterol or just be something that runs in the family.

If you have high cholesterol you can do lots of things to reduce it, so seek advice from your GP.

Lasers can be used to burn out the yellowy fat. They usually disappear for good, especially if your cholesterol is normal. You can get them cut out but this leaves a little scar. Both methods are a bit sore, so opt for a local anaesthetic.

Cost: Expect to pay around £500+ per session.

Patient pain rating: 6–7 (1–10, 1=pain-free)

Treatment time: 30–60 minutes per session

How long do they last? The fat deposits disappear but they may return if your cholesterol remains high.

Lasers for pearly bumps

Little rounded pearly lumps, called syringomas, under the eyes and on the cheeks are benign tumours of the sweat glands. They are usually a cosmetic problem rather than a danger. I recently removed some of these for an actor patient of mine because he was worried they would show up on screen. But you should get them checked by a dermatologist to be extra sure.

I use lasers with a little anaesthetic to flatten off syringomas. This works well, but two to three sessions are required and some may need retreating.

Cost: Expect to pay around £500 per session.
Patient pain rating: 6–7 (1–10, 1=pain-free)
Treatment time: 45–60 minutes per session
(can take 2–3 sessions)
How long does it last? Effects last 2–3 years but they may recur.

Lightening dark patches

If you have dark or black skin and darker patches near your eyes, this uneven pigment is probably the result of sun damage, but sometimes it is triggered by skin conditions such as acne, eczema or dermatitis. Protect yourself from the sun to stop the cells from producing more pigment and get a lightening agent from any chemist. These lotions help to slow down the production of more pigment.

The best no-surgery treatment involves a two-pronged attack: firstly, a powerful medical prescription-only lightening agent, which patients apply at home; secondly, a course of gentle chemical peels done at the clinic. The chemical peel bleaches and removes the pigmentation from the top layers of skin while the lightening agent slows down the development of more pigment in the under-layers.

Cost: £50 for a tube of strong lightening agent from a cosmetic doctor. £75–£100 per session for a light chemical peel.

Patient pain rating: 2–3 (1–10, 1=pain-free)

Treatment time: 15 minutes

How long does it last? Effects can be maintained with a session every 2–3 months, or when you feel it is necessary, and by applying the cream one month on and then one month off.

No-Surgery Treatments
for Lips

For girls, lips are an important element of the look. Mouths are part of that facial triangle of attraction that people focus on when they first meet, so lips are second only to eyes when it comes to the amount of attention they get from admirers. The anthropologist Desmond Morris points out that women's lips are sexy because they mimic the genital area. Enhancing lip definition, colour and shape will boost the effectiveness of these important assets.

I find many girls are extra nervous about getting their lips 'done' because of the disaster stories they have read in the press. However, these disasters are avoidable – it is simply a matter of using the right filler and getting a qualified practitioner to do the job. If you follow my tips and advice, it won't happen to you.

Common problems

☆ thinning lips and lost definition

☆ pouts

☆ small lips

☆ downturned mouth

☆ smile lines

☆ pucker lines (especially if you have smoked)

☆ the mask of pregnancy across the top lip (see also Chins)

☆ hair on upper lip (see also the chapter on Anywhere)

Filling a downturned smile

I see some relatively young patients for whom a downturned mouth is hereditary, but the majority are in their forties and upwards, whose mouths have turned down over time. Using a bit of filler we can make a sulky mouth straight. Not upturned – we don't want to make it lift up like Jack Nicholson's penguin.

With a touch of filler in the corner of the lip line, a little on the top lip and a bit more in the marionette line (the groove that goes down towards the jaw) I can really lift the face. It creates a more contented, smiley look.

By smile lines I mean the undesirable ones that become a fixed wrinkle, not the desirable ones that come and go – we want to keep those! This can happen more on one side, or you can get several lining up, which we call primary and secondary smile lines. How you sleep or any dental problems you have, creating a bit of asymmetry in your face, can bring these on, but a bit of filler can lift them out. I'm also hopeful that radiofrequency will prove helpful here, by tightening the skin to stretch out the wrinkle.

Cost: £350 per session.
Patient pain rating: 3–4 with an anaesthetic (1–10, 1=pain-free)
Treatment time: 15 minutes
How long does it last? 5–6 months (longer for some)

Reviving lips using fillers

Our lips look thinner as time goes by. This loss of volume in the pink part of the lip starts to show when collagen production slows down – usually from the late thirties onwards. Your lips will probably lose plumpness sooner if you are a regular smoker, because collagen breakdown is boosted by smoking.

Fillers are great for replacing a bit of lost volume. Very gently increasing the fullness of the lips and filling in lines can really transform the look of the face. This is one of my favourite treatments – I think it looks great.

Some doctors decide not to use an anaesthetic because anaesthetics slightly alter the shape of the lips and they would rather be able to see the original. But filler injections are quite painful and in between injections the doctor needs to massage your lips, smoothing out any little blobs so you don't get lumpy bits. This is difficult when it inflicts pain on your poor patient. So I just take a Polaroid before I start and work from the picture. I find the positives override the negatives.

☆ *Tips*

☆ Always make sure your doctor gives you a dental block. It is not just your comfort I'm thinking of – it helps the doctor to do a better job too.

☆ If you are a first-timer, get the doctor to be conservative to start with and then leave it a month before deciding whether you need more. Agree a price for this beforehand. You can't take filler out!

☆ When you first look in the mirror after you have had the treatment, be prepared: it looks dramatic initially. This is the swelling, which goes down after a few days.

☆ Fillers can bring on cold sores, so if you are prone, use one of the preventative creams or tablets available from chemists as an insurance policy. Use them for one day before your treatment and then for a week after it.

☆ Don't fix up special events for the following day: most patients get swelling for one to two days, and for some it is seven to ten days.

☆ Keep massaging the treated area three times a day for a week, to avoid getting lumps.

☆ For a good natural result, seek an experienced practitioner: one who will respect the natural shape of your lips. Remember it is not easy to change the lip shape, it is the volume you are increasing. Permanent pouts require surgery, and the downside is that as the rest of your face changes with time, your lips will look out of place.

Cost: £350 per session, depending on how much filler you need.
Patient pain rating: 2–3 with an anaesthetic (1–10, 1=pain-free)
Treatment time: 15 minutes
How long does it last? 5–6 months (up to a year for some)

Creating a pout using fillers

This is a different treatment. The desire for a pout is a cyclical thing – a fashion that comes and goes. If you are a younger woman wanting a pout but your lips are naturally thin and your mouth small, fillers can't give you a mouth like Liz Hurley. It is easy to accentuate the existing outline, but I find that trying to change the lip shape with filler doesn't usually work well. It looks great on a few, but on most it looks obvious and unnatural. Think 'accentuate' rather than 'change', and talk about your expectations with your cosmetic doctor.

Cost: £350 per session depending on how much filler you need.
Patient pain rating: 2–3 with an anaesthetic (1–10, 1=pain-free)
Treatment time: 15 minutes
How long does it last? 5–6 months (up to 8 months for some)

The truth about Leslie Ash

Leslie Ash was very unfortunate. She had a new type of filler, designed to last longer. Most fillers contain hyaluronic acid, which lasts around five to six months (slightly less for the pout look), but the filler Leslie Ash received had a mixture of hyaluronic acid and permanent granules. The granules were added to make the filler permanent, but they trigger an allergic reaction in some people (swelling and sometimes lumpiness too). Tragically, this was the case with the lovely Leslie Ash, and because the filler is designed to last a long time and you can't take it out, she's stuck with this for several years.

A few women have come to me like this, asking if I can sort out a reaction they have had to a long-lasting filler, but in these situations all I can do is inject them with steroids to reduce the reaction. This can be successful, but unfortunately in Leslie Ash's case it doesn't seem to have been.

The moral

Just because something is 'new' it doesn't mean it is better. Be wary of any new products that come on to the market claiming to last longer. Even if they work well, implanting something in your lips that lasts a long time will end up looking obvious and incongruous as the rest of your face changes with time. I think hyaluronic fillers are excellent and safe. The fact that they don't last as long is less of an inconvenience than an allergy. I expect Leslie Ash would agree.

Fillers for pucker lines

The edges of your lips and your cupid's bow lose definition as you get older.

A bit of lipstick and liner can do the trick, but if you have vertical lip lines, makeup tends to bleed into them. Lip lines are part of natural ageing, but whether you get them and how many you get are determined by hereditary factors and whether you have smoked. The shape of your jaw and teeth can play a role too – the more set back they are, the less they support the skin around the mouth, making it more susceptible to creasing and shrinkage.

Hyaluronic fillers are good for filling in these lines. The effects last up to four months if you smoke and six months if you don't. Massaging is particularly important because the movement when you eat and talk can shift the filler and give you lumps. Massage the skin around your mouth three times a day for seven to ten days after the treatment and you will be fine.

☆ *Tips*

- ☆ Stay off the fags – inhaling chemicals that hasten collagen breakdown will leave your mouth badly lined.
- ☆ Remember to moisturize and balm with sun protection. The dryer your lips are the more they shrivel and crease.
- ☆ Some balms can temporarily plump lips a little.
- ☆ Once you have had the treatment, use your lipstick and liner to enhance the definition. Semi-permanent makeup can look good.

Cost: £350 per session.
Patient pain rating: 3–4 with an anaesthetic (1–10, 1=pain-free)
Treatment time: 15 minutes
How long does it last? 4–6 months

On semi-permanent makeup

This area of cosmetics is not regulated, so either go on a recommendation or be sure to examine your practitioner's portfolio before you commit to a treatment. Ask if the pigments they use meet health and safety standards. The effects usually last about a year and cost upwards of £500.

Lasers for smoker's lines

This is a more radical approach that involves a period of recovery before you see the result, but the results last longer. It is good for severe lines like those due to smoking. Very carefully, a strong laser removes the wrinkled skin around the mouth, a little bit at a time, which also stimulates the production of new unwrinkled skin.

You have a dental block for this treatment, so it doesn't hurt, but it can be quite uncomfortable for the next couple of days. Then it starts to settle down and after two weeks you will be out and about with a bit of makeup on. Four to six months later, the skin will be back to normal and you can enjoy the effects for up to five years. Sometimes it makes the skin look a bit pale, but this doesn't seem to bother my patients. They are usually pretty pleased with the outcome.

☆ *Tips*

- ☆ Get the doctor to prescribe some strong painkillers for the first few days.
- ☆ Be prepared for what feels like very bad sunburn.
- ☆ You won't want to go out for a couple of weeks, so organize yourself: take some time out and decline invites to key social events.
- ☆ This is a one-off treatment – not to be repeated.

Cost: £1,300 per session (usually one session only).
Patient pain rating: 6–9, not during the treatment but for a few days after it (1–10, 1=pain-free)
Treatment time: 45 minutes
How long does it last? Up to 5 years.

Botox for smoker's lines

If doctors offer you botox for this, be warned: the distance between a good result and a problem is very narrow. A small error can temporarily impede your ability to enunciate or whistle. I would only consider doing this on a patient with a real sucking-lemons mouth, but in general I avoid it because of the possible side-effects.

Cost: Expect to pay £250–£300 per session.
Patient pain rating: 2–3 (1–10, 1=pain-free)
Treatment time: 10 minutes
How long does it last? 3–4 months

On severe smoker's lines and dermabrasion

I don't offer this treatment as lasers have taken over now.
Dermabrasion machines are outdated – they are like
Black & Decker drills with wire brushes attached. A few
surgeons still use this on facelift patients because a facelift
alone doesn't improve the wrinkles around the mouth, but
it is only performed while a facelift patient is still under
anaesthetic. Lasers are a more accurate way of de-wrinkling
this area and this can be carried out under a local
anaesthetic.

**Note: Dermabrasion and microdermabrasion are not
the same!** They both remove surface layers of skin but by
completely different means. Microdermabrasion is a gentle
process that gets results over time via repeated treatments.

No-Surgery Treatments for *Cheeks*

There is another facial triangle of attraction, apart from the one made by your mouth and eyes. The temples of the forehead are the upper corners and the cheeks guide the onlooker's eye down towards the third corner, which is the chin. When we are young this clearly defined triangle makes us look attractive, but unfortunately it doesn't stay like this. Want to know why?

Over time, our cheeks lose plumpness because some of the fat and collagen disappears, and the fat that remains moves downwards. It moves beyond the jaw line, so the chin loses its prominence; thus, the triangle of attraction becomes less defined. However, by using no-surgery treatments to soften curves and tighten any saggy bits we can replace the lost volume in the cheeks and redefine the jaw line to get that triangular emphasis back again – we can make you look younger.

The complexion is important too. Any blemishes, sun damage, scars and uneven colouring are difficult to conceal on the cheeks, which makes people self-conscious. No-surgery treatments can be used to reduce scarring, even out skin tone, restore a healthy glow, remove broken veins, reduce lines and fade sun spots. These improvements can really restore a patient's confidence, and for some it is a life-changing difference, particularly if you suffer from acne.

Common problems

- ☆ fat pads
- ☆ flushing and redness from acne rosacea
- ☆ nose-to-lip lines
- ☆ acne scars or scars from surgery or injury
- ☆ hollow cheeks
- ☆ sun spots (see also the chapter on Anywhere)
- ☆ the mask of pregnancy (see also the chapter on Chins)

IPL for little broken veins

These appear as red dots where a tiny blood vessel has been damaged. This can happen with rosacea and weathering, or when the skin is a bit dry and gets knocked, or a small cut gets a bit infected. IPL is the treatment for these.

Cost: Expect to pay £200 per session.

Patient pain rating: 5 (1–10, 1=pain-free)

Treatment time: 5–30 mins per session

How long does it last? Permanently, but you may need a couple of sessions to get any that you didn't catch the first time.

Reducing fat pads

These are pads of fat that sit on the top of the cheekbone, just below the eye. They are usually small, roughly 1.5 cm long and sausage-shaped. Patients don't like the way these pads make them look tired or heavy-eyed.

A lot of people have them but they sit unobtrusively, amongst youthful cheek fat, until, with time and gravity, the covering fat moves down to expose them. I see these on women in their forties and above. They are more noticeable on thinner faces because there is less fat covering them. They are stubborn little things: they don't get removed in facelifts or eye-bag surgery. Sometimes people come to see me after a facelift because their fat pads are still there, and having a facelift can even make them more obvious.

Liposuction

It's possible to remove fat pads with liposuction using fine needles, but it is not the ideal treatment because you will inevitably get a small scar. Facelifts and eye-bag surgery also leave small scars behind, but on other parts of the face the surgeon can hide the scar in a crease. Cheeks offer no such hiding places. You need a local anaesthetic for fat-pad liposuction and you will be swollen and bruised for a couple of weeks after the treatment.

Cost: £1,000 per session – you may need up to 3 sessions.
Patient pain rating: 4–5 post treatment, due to swelling and bruising (1–10, 1=pain-free)
Treatment time: 10 minutes each side
How long does it last? Permanently

Radiofrequency

I'm hopeful that radiofrequency will be the answer for patients with this problem. We know radiofrequency can be used to tighten the skin, but there is also good anecdotal evidence to show that we can use it to break down fat cells too. This treatment is still evolving; no proper studies have been done yet, but it is a very interesting development. Keep an eye on my website for updates. I expect it will cost around £300–£400 per session and might take up to 4 sessions 4 weeks apart to dissolve them completely.

☆ Tip

☆ These radiofrequency machines are very new. Depending on where you live, you may need to travel quite a distance to get to a practitioner who has one. But this will change as clinics respond to demand.

IPL for excessive flushing

This mostly affects women, usually in their thirties and
upwards. It is four times more common in women than
men and typically starts with redness on the tip of the nose,
which eventually spreads to the cheeks, chin, the centre of
the forehead and between the eyebrows.

A change in temperature, a boozy drink or spicy food can
all cause uncomfortable flushes if you have rosacea. After a
while, flaky skin, red spots and visible red blood vessels
develop within the red area and it slowly spreads. In chronic
cases, sufferers get a lumpy red and blue nose. This is the
end stage of rosacea and unfortunately it makes the patient
look like an alcoholic. Occasionally, rosacea affects eyes,
making them red and sore, in which case you should
consult an eye specialist. We don't know what causes rosacea
and there isn't a cure, but in most cases it comes and goes
until eventually it burns itself out.

☆ *Tips*

- ☆ On a hot date but don't want a hot flush? Avoid boozy drinks
  and don't order the chilli.
- ☆ Similarly, don't meet after a sauna or a winter jog in the park
  if you want to make a good impression – changes in
  temperature make flushes worse.

☆ When you change your makeup, patch-test it for a few days to ensure it doesn't make your redness worse.

☆ Use vitamin E, as it is anti-inflammatory.

☆ A vitamin C lotion will help reduce redness, but test it first before you apply it thoroughly, to ensure it doesn't make your cheeks flare up.

☆ Ensure your practitioner's IPL machine has a cooling device.

☆ Don't have an IPL treatment when you are tanned or flushed because the machine recognizes rosacea by its colour, so if your whole face is colourful it will get confused and heat up everything.

Cost: £250 per session with 2–3 maintenance sessions a year.

Patient pain rating: 4–5 with a cooling device (1–10, 1=pain-free)

Treatment time: 15 minutes per session

How long does it last? 1–4 months – it varies between patients.

Filling in nose-to-lip lines

Two small ligaments, a bit like taut pieces of string, run from the base of your nose out towards the corners of your mouth. As we get older, cheek fat moves down, gets caught on them and folds over, forming nose-to-lip lines. How obvious, deep or long they are varies between individuals. They are a genetically determined thing and are often deeper on one side, or more obvious if you have lost or gained a lot of weight.

Lifting these lines using hyaluronic fillers is one of the most common treatments I do. I don't remove them completely, I just soften them. They are normal lines of definition in the face so we don't want to remove them.

You could get a surgeon to extract fat from another part of you – usually your bottom – and inject this under the line instead of filler. However, I wouldn't recommend this treatment: you will be swollen for up to four weeks, it can end up looking uneven, and you've no argument if you get accused of talking out of your bottom!

 Tips

☆ An unequal bite makes this worse. If you have one, ask your dentist what can be done. Having your teeth fixed can stop nose-to-lip lines getting worse and any filler treatment you have will last longer.

☆ Don't blow up balloons, play the trumpet or chew gum for at least 1– 2 weeks after the treatment – excessive movement could shift the filler about and make it set unevenly.

☆ Massage, massage, massage: three times a day for one week, to prevent lumps.

☆ Perlane and Restylane are safe hyaluronic acid fillers.

☆ Sculptra is a good filler for deeper folds and the same price as hyaluronic acid, so you get more filler for your money.

Cost: Expect to pay £350 – £700 per session, depending on how much filler you require.

Patient pain rating: 3–4 with an anaesthetic

Treatment time: 15 minutes

How long does it last? 9–12 months

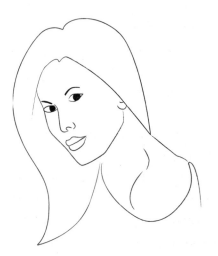

Filling & defining cheeks

Weight loss is often the cause, but, for most, hollow cheeks come about through the natural loss of facial fat that happens with age. For some, however, it is a condition known as lipodystrophy, which is either passed on genetically, or, for those receiving treatment for AIDS, it is a side-effect of the drugs they have to take, which dissolve cheek fat, making the patient's face emaciated.

However, you can replace lost cheek fat with filler. This usually takes two to three sessions because, to achieve a smooth shape, the practitioner needs to build up the filler in layers, allowing each layer to set in between sessions. The last session is usually just a bit of fine-tuning.

By putting a bit of filler on top of the cheekbones, where the fat has disappeared, you can really alter the shape of the face – if it is appropriate – but you need an experienced cosmetic doctor to do this for you. For example, a very square jaw line can look much softer by enhancing the cheeks. Sculptra is a good filler for this. It is a thicker consistency, so you get more filler for your money. It lasts for over a year, but you will need top-ups from time to time.

To help me work out where to put the filler, I look at the patient's face from behind at an angle, to examine what is called the ogee curve. That is the wavy pattern made by the outward curve of the cheekbone flowing into the inward curve of the cheek hollow. I look for where it seems flat to determine where to put the filler. A more curvaceous ogee enhances the shape of the face.

☆ *Tips:*

☆ Clear your social diary – after treatment the face normally looks swollen for several days.

☆ Massage, massage, massage if you don't want your cheeks to look lumpy. Three times a day for the first three weeks following each treatment.

Cost: Expect to pay £300 to £600 per session, depending on how much filler you need.

Patient pain rating: 4–5 (1–10, 1=pain-free)

Treatment time: 15–30 minutes per session

How long does it last? Over 12 months

Reducing nose-to-lip lines

Radiofrequency remodelling can be used to tighten the skin, which in turn gives the cheek a bit of a lift, leaving less skin folding over the nose-to-lip line. You could combine this treatment with fillers for extra effect. One treatment of 45 minutes can be enough, but for most it takes three to four goes, spaced two to four weeks apart. It is a very new treatment in the UK, but because it has been in use in the US (and other countries) for a couple of years now, we have evidence that it works. Expect to see up to a 20 per cent improvement immediately, and more during the six months following treatment. On some parts of the face this treatment can feel uncomfortably hot, but less so on the cheeks because the cheek fat absorbs some of the heat.

Cost: This will change and vary from doctor to doctor depending on the type of machine they have. There is a big variation, anything from £500 to £3,500 per session, and you may need 3–4 sessions four weeks apart.

Patient pain rating: 4–5, although it varies between machines and different parts of the face (1–10, 1=pain-free)

Treatment time: 45 minutes

How long does it last? Up to 2 years, as far as we know – it may last even longer.

Acne

Who gets acne?

According to the statistics, 90 per cent of us will experience some form of acne during our lives. More people are getting it and adult acne is increasingly common in women in their thirties and forties. No one knows why. We know hormones play a part but we don't know exactly how. The worst sufferers usually have thicker, greasier skin and the grease itself is of a heavier consistency. In a mild case of acne, the cells lining each skin pore tend to be bigger, forming narrower exits, so the pores are more easily blocked. When a few dead skin cells get stuck in the exit, causing a blockage, you get a blackhead or a whitehead. The only difference between these two is the blackhead has a bit of pigment in it – it is not dirt.

Acne sufferers also have bacteria in their skin that under normal circumstances don't cause any trouble; but when a pore gets blocked and the warm, sealed, stagnant environment inside the pore makes these bacteria breed like wildfire, and the bacteria love it. As they multiply, you get a build-up of pus that swells the skin.

If nothing happens the pus breaks the skin, escapes and get washed away – but most people don't wait, they pick. The pus can also be washed away by the immune system. But in very severe cases it forms an acne cyst: a lump under the skin that is bigger than the spot and hangs around for a lot longer.

To squeeze or not to squeeze?

If your spot is sore or red, don't pick it. What you see on the surface is the tip of the iceberg. Some may come out, but some may also go deeper in, causing a cyst, which is worse.

If you have a non-infected blackhead or whitehead you can give it a bit of a steam and use a blackhead extractor (available from chemists) to squeeze out the blockage. Your nails tend to be a bit sharp, but if that is all you have to hand then please be gentle and cover them with a clean tissue so they don't damage the skin.

Treating a mild case of acne

☆ Exfoliate regularly to help prevent grease glands clogging.

☆ Avoid heavy creams because they can clog up the grease glands more.

☆ Eat a healthy, balanced diet. Not because some food gives you spots but because the immune system will then be more efficient to deal with a low-grade infection in the skin. Arm your immune system with the power to do its job.

☆ Try an over-the-counter lotion or potion containing benzoyl peroxide. This ingredient kills the bacteria by blasting it with oxygen. It might make your skin a bit dry and red and it doesn't penetrate deeply, but it can help to control the zits.

☆ Be sure your handbag staples include a lotion or potion containing glycolic acid. This ingredient is an anti-inflammatory so it will reduce some of the redness and make the spot(s) less noticeable.

☆ Emergencies only: wet the spot and dab an aspirin on it. Aspirin is an anti-inflammatory that can tone down the redness, but it is less efficient than a cream made for the purpose.

Myth: A bit of sun will heal up your acne

Acne sufferers say sun heals up their spots, and twenty years ago acne sufferers were given sunlamp treatment. We now know this actually makes acne worse (and damages the skin!). What happens is known as 'the Majorca flare'. Your spots improve when you are in the sun, but then the skin cells thicken to protect you from the sun. So, when you come back, those thick cells around the pores make the openings narrower so they get blocked more easily.

Myth: Chocolate, cheese and chips cause spots

No. There is no evidence that this is true, but if you only eat chocolate, cheese and chips then you are getting an imbalanced diet, and an imbalanced diet can make acne worse.

Treating acne using lasers

An acne laser is a laser similar to blue light in that it also kills the special bacteria that live in acne-prone skin. It does seem to help a little bit with acne. There are some studies to show it works and some very limited evidence that it improves acne scars, but I take the view that firing lasers into teenagers is not a good idea until we know more about the long-term consequences. This is true of all lasers. As a rule, we don't use lasers on young kids while their skin is still developing – with one exception, and that is for birthmarks. I use a gentler blue-light alternative for younger acne patients. The developers of lasers for acne also claim that they stimulate skin rejuvenation, but this is still up for argument.

Cost: £300+ per session. May take 3 or more sessions.
Patient pain rating: 3–4 (1–10, 1=pain-free)
Treatment time: 30 minutes
How long does it last? It is not a cure, so maintenance treatments are needed every 4–6 months.

Treating acne with blue light

Blue light can reach the bacteria under the skin and kill it without damaging the surface. Blue light won't necessarily cure acne, but most of my patients see considerable improvement and find a series of treatments from time to time helps keep it at bay. It is quite comfortable to have and it doesn't cause dryness or soreness like some on-the-skin treatments.

Expect your spots to get a bit worse at first. This is normal (there is more about this in Part Two). By about four to six weeks you should start to see a change for the better. Between 70 and 80 per cent of people will get an improvement with this treatment, the extent of which varies between 10 and 90 per cent.

Cost: £350 for a course of 8 sessions, 2 per week, for 4 weeks.
Patient pain rating: 1 (1– 10, 1=pain-free)
Treatment time: 30 minutes
How long does it last? This is a maintenance programme. It varies from person to person, but the benefits can last up to 6 months.

Swallowed acne treatments

A low dose of antibiotic from a GP or a clinic can help kill off the bacterial infection. For women who have a hormone imbalance, hormone tablets like the contraceptive pill (Dianette, or Yasmin, are the most common) work by balancing out the male and female hormones. You only need a tiny hormonal shift to reduce the problem.

Roaccutane is a formulation of vitamin A. Sadly, it has had bad press – in a few cases the families of children who took their own lives claim Roaccutane was to blame. There are a small number of cases but these were widely reported. There is no way of knowing whether it was the drug or depression about their affliction that made them commit suicide.

The negativity surrounding this drug is a shame, because it really is the only proven cure for acne. It has an 80 per cent success rate and I've seen it change people's lives. You need to take it under hospital supervision and to use contraception because it is known to cause foetal deformities. The treatment takes three months and you may need a second course, but it is pretty effective.

Tip

☆ Roaccutane is very expensive to have privately, so go to your
GP who can refer you to a consultant dermatologist. This is
the only way you can get Roaccutane in the UK.

Cost: If you were to go privately, expect to pay £1,000 for a course
of treatment, which includes doctor's fee and blood tests.

Patient pain rating: 1–2 – that's for the blood tests you have
before and during the treatments (1–10, 1=pain-free)

Treatment time: A minimum of 3 months, and some require
more than one course.

How long does it last? Can give a permanent cure.

Self-applied acne treatments

Other than topical antibiotics, which are available on prescription from a GP, clinic or dermatologist, Retin-A, a form of vitamin A, can unplug the blackheads and whiteheads and reduce inflammation. There are a variety of vitamin A-based potions around, but the strength you need to make an impact on acne is only available on prescription, so ask a GP, cosmetic doctor or dermatologist. A gel form is preferable to a cream because you don't want extra grease on your skin.

Retin-A is available to acne sufferers on the NHS. Otherwise, you can purchase some from a private clinic or your cosmetic doctor for about £50.

Light peels also unblock grease glands to reduce blackheads and whiteheads, and because they contain anti-inflammatory ingredients they have the added advantage of reducing zits and softening scars. You need one and sometimes two courses of six peels, with a month between each peel, to get the best results. You wouldn't see much of a difference if you just had one. Once you are happy with the results you just need maintenance treatments every two to three months.

Cost: £250 for a course of 6, you may need more than one course.
Patient pain rating: 1 (1– 10, 1=pain-free)
Treatment time: 30 minutes
How long does it last? This is more a matter of ongoing maintenance.

No-Surgery Treatments for the Nose

People who have a problem with their nose are usually unhappy with its size, shape or colour. The male ideal is a longer, more distinctive nose, and for the female it is a more petite nose, according to research carried out by the psychologist Bernhard Fink. To radically reshape and resize a nose requires a surgeon, an anaesthetist and an overnight stay in hospital, but we can make minor corrections to nose shape with no-surgery treatments. We can also sort out a few other things that make people self-conscious, like redness, moles, little blood vessels that have popped up on the skin and straying hair.

Common problems

- ☆ asymmetrical nose
- ☆ droopy nose
- ☆ veins
- ☆ enlarged, red, lumpy-bumpy nose (end-stage of acne rosacea)
- ☆ hairy nose

Fillers for deviated noses

Changing nose shape usually requires surgery, but if you only have a minor deviation we can lift out a kink with some filler and get a good result. By a minor deviation I mean the nose looks slightly asymmetrical – a bit crooked from the front view, or a little dip when you look from the side. We do this for people who have banged their noses – small breaks or chips rather than a major rugby injury – and others whose noses are naturally uneven. This takes 15 minutes, some hyaluronic fillers, some anaesthetic cream and an experienced cosmetic doctor.

☆ *Tip*

☆ As with all fillers, make sure you massage the area for at least three weeks after treatment.

Cost: £200–£400 per session, depending on the amount of filler.
Patient pain rating: 5 (1–10, 1=pain-free)
Treatment time: 15 minutes
How long does it last? Up to a year.

Lifting a droopy nose

Noses get a bit longer as we age. Inside your nose you have got bone at the top and cartilage at the bottom, and it is the cartilage bit that droops down and widens with age. Patients who come in for this treatment don't like the shape – the way it bends over at the end. We can perk up a droopy nose by putting a bit of filler in the nasal septum to raise the tip. This is a subtle improvement – we get more obvious enhancement when we straighten out kinks on the top part of the nose.

Cost: £200– £400 per session, depending on the amount of filler.
Patient pain rating: 5 (1–10, 1=pain-free)
Treatment time: 15 minutes
How long does it last? Up to a year.

Removing obvious veins

Fine pink and purple veins are signs of weathering from exposure to the elements, hot or cold, and we can be genetically predisposed to these. They can pop up anywhere, but a lot of people get these somewhere on their nose: the bridge, side, tip, or the visible bit of the nostrils. A tendency for these little red veins typically goes hand in hand with a skin condition like rosacea or eczema, and nose surgery causes them too, because straightening the cartilage interferes with the blood supply. Whatever the cause, veins like these can be lasered out quite easily.

☆ *Tip*

☆ If you get these little veins, make sure your daily moisturizer or makeup contains a sunscreen, and don't forget to put it on your nose. This will help prevent new ones.

Cost: Expect to pay £200 per session.
Patient pain rating: 3–4 (1–10, 1=pain-free)
Treatment time: 15 minutes
How long do they last? They usually go, but if you get new ones you will need to go back for maintenance sessions.

Lasers for red bumpy noses

A permanently red lumpy-bumpy nose (rhinophyma) is a symptom of long-term rosacea. We can smooth it off and get rid of the lumpiness with a laser, carefully removing the damaged skin, tiny bit by tiny bit, in a safe and controlled way.

As it is difficult and painful to inject a local anaesthetic in the nose so we use a cream anaesthetic, which isn't as effective so this treatment is sore and involves a bit of recovery time. However, I find patients who want rid of their lumpy-bumpy nose are happy to put up with a bit of discomfort because they are determined to sort it out. The worst of the soreness lasts for a couple of days, but you can take painkillers. By week three it will feel normal again. During these three weeks you have to keep bathing it and putting Vaseline on to stop the air getting to it. This way it doesn't scab, and the skin heals with a smooth finish. Your nose will look red for three to six months but you can camouflage it, and when the redness goes it looks good and the results are permanent, as long as you keep your rosacea under control.

Cost: £1,300 per session (you may need two sessions).
Patient pain rating: 8–9 after the anaesthetic has worn off
Treatment time: 15 minutes
How long does it last? Long-term

Removing unwanted hair using IPL or lasers

It is not exclusively men who have unruly nasal hair. Some women discover stray hair on their noses – not just coming out of their nostrils, but also from the bridge and the tip. This can be hereditary but it is more often a symptom of hormone imbalance. Nine per cent of women suffer from low oestrogen, which can also bring about acne, obesity, infertility and ovarian cysts. Sometimes a hormone imbalance is a side-effect of drugs: hormonal drugs (obtained illegally) to improve their sex drives, or steroids for bodybuilding.

I once saw a professional lady bodybuilder who had this problem because she had been on testosterone for years. Even when she stopped taking the hormone, the hair continued to grow. This woman had to shave her face twice a day. She had hair in all the places men have hair. Years of bodybuilding drugs turned the hair follicles on permanently and made them so resilient that whatever we did to get rid of them, they just grew back.

Generally speaking, however, a hairy nose is more often a treatment we do for men. You girls aren't the only ones with beauty worries. As men get older we lose hair on our heads and it springs out of our nostrils, nose and ears. So keep this one up your sleeve in case you need it for the man in your life.

IPL and lasers work in the same way; they both destroy the hair follicle. You will need up to four sessions to catch all the hairs because of the way hair grows in cycles (see the section on Lasers in Part Two). After that your hair should stay away, and if any do come back they will be much finer, not coarse and dark.

 Tips

☆ If it is only a few hairs you want removed – less than ten – electrolysis will work out less expensive.

☆ Testosterone makes hair more virulent, so with men there is a 50:50 chance the hair will grow back within six months. If it does, you will need this treatment yearly to keep the problem under control.

☆ These machines have only been around for eight or nine years, so although the US authorities have decided that permanent means hairs not regrowing after three cycles, I prefer to say long-term until we can be sure.

☆ IPL doesn't work well on tanned skin, so this is a good treatment to have in the winter.

☆ If you are dark-skinned, choose lasers rather than IPL.

Cost: Expect to pay £75 per session.

Patient pain rating: 3–4 for women and 10 for men – not that it hurts men more, but everything is 10 for men! (1–10, 1=pain-free)

Treatment time: 5 minutes

How long does it last? Can be a couple of years or more.

Myth: Shaving makes hair grow back stronger

This is a fallacy. Neither plucking nor shaving changes the nature of the hair that grows back. I'd shave if I were you – it is less painful.

No-Surgery Treatments
for the
Forehead

The skin on our foreheads is relatively thick and well greased, which provides more protection from fine ageing lines. Here, the uninvited guests are more usually expression lines – the imprints of frowning and raising our eyebrows. This is where botox can work a little magic.

There are several no-surgery treatments for evening out the skin tone and texture on our foreheads. Whether it is broken veins and patches of sun spots – common here because foreheads face sunwards – or a problem with spots due to the extra grease in this area, there are lots of things we can do.

Common problems

- ☆ wrinkles and frown-lines
- ☆ large pores
- ☆ enlarged grease glands
- ☆ blackheads, whiteheads and milia (pronounced mill-ia)
- ☆ lipomas and cysts
- ☆ sun spots and spider naevi (see also the chapter on Anywhere)
- ☆ the mask of pregnancy (see also the chapter on Chins)

Filling in wrinkles & lines

Lifting out the frown furrow with filler works well, but it makes sense to combine this with botox to stop more lines developing. However, fillers don't work so well for horizontal lines. This is because the skin on the forehead has bone directly underneath it and less soft tissue to cushion it, which means fillers sometimes look uneven. Less is more if you are treating worry-lines with filler. It is better to treat these with botox before they become well established.

Cost: Expect to pay £350 per session.
Patient pain rating: 3–4 with an anaesthetic (1–10, 1=pain-free)
Treatment time: 15 minutes
How long does it last? 6–9 months

Botox for frown-lines

No one welcomes the onset of 'frown' lines, the vertical lines between the eyebrows. They complain about looking overly serious, stern, worried or even angry, when in actual fact they feel fine. Worry-lines are just as unpopular. These run horizontally and they are reinforced when you frown, look up, or raise your eyebrows, and when you make a look of surprise or concern. And women in particular tend to subconsciously raise their eyebrows more, to achieve an open-eyed look. Men don't seem to do this, maybe because heavy eyes are considered an attractive feature on men.

Nugget

People who suffer facial paralysis due to strokes or Bell's Palsy don't get wrinkles because they can't make the expressions responsible for forming them.

Botox is by far the best treatment for horizontal lines. Injected into the muscles in the forehead (not into the lines themselves), botox makes it harder to raise your eyebrows high enough to push the forehead skin up into pleats. If you have botox before your frown-lines or worry-lines become deep, this will be enough to prevent them and make the early signs disappear because you are no longer reinforcing them. If furrows are deeply established already, botox will soften them but you will probably need a bit of filler as well, to lift out the crease.

There is no optimum age for treating them. They appear sooner in people who naturally have more expressive faces or fair, sun-damaged skin that wrinkles early. A good number of my patients come to me in their mid to late twenties and they have found botox has been a good preventive treatment for them.

Myth: I will be left expressionless

No, unless you see a practitioner who is not properly trained. Botox just works on the muscles where it is injected. It can't float around freezing other muscles in your face.

Cost: Expect to pay £250–£300 per session.
Patient pain rating: 2–3 (1–10, 1=pain-free)
Treatment time: 10 minutes
How long does it last? 3–4 months

☆ *Tips*

☆ Ignore products that boast they can 'do away' with either vertical or horizontal lines – these claims are based on wishful thinking, not scientific proof.

☆ Good skincare is important if you want to delay the arrival of forehead lines, and essential if you are investing in professional treatments such as botox and fillers. Don't let your skin dry out, and feed it all the vitamins it needs to repair and renew itself. Eat a varied diet and read my chapter on lotions and potions for advice on how to feed it from the outside.

On large pores

People talk about large pores when what they are really referring to are open grease glands. Strictly speaking, a pore is the exit of a sweat gland that isn't visible to the naked eye. Some people just have naturally large open grease glands, but most people's grease glands get larger as they get older because they elongate as the skin becomes less elastic over time.

What you can do

Not much can be done about enlarged pores, although exfoliating regularly with a fruit or salicylic-acid-based gel will give them a good clear-out, which makes them shrink slightly and look less obvious. If you have greasy or oily skin, make sure you use a gel or lotion rather than a cream, which tends to clog them up and give you whiteheads and blackheads.

The clinical treatment for this problem is to clear out the enlarged skin pores using a light chemical peel, but this is an ongoing process because they will re-clog after two to four weeks. The effect of the peel can be prolonged by the use of an exfoliator at home, but check with your therapist before you start.

☆ Tip

☆ Ignore products that claim to reduce large pores. I don't know of anything that can do this.

Cost: Expect to pay £75 per session every 4–8 weeks.
Patient pain rating: 2 (1–10, 1=pain-free)
Treatment time: 30 minutes
How long does it last? 1–2 months

Enlarged grease glands

These look like yellow craters, a raised edge with a hole in the middle, and they are pretty common in people of 30 and upwards. A grease gland swells up into a hard little bump because, for reasons unknown, it goes into overdrive and produces too many grease cells. Although this isn't a serious condition, don't get your nail scissors out and start tackling it yourself if you would rather avoid an infection and the possibility of scarring.

We can destroy the spot layer by layer using a laser, or scrape it off in layers using a curette (a little instrument that looks like a tiny melon scoop). Enlarged grease glands can also be frozen or cauterized. All these techniques must be carried out by a cosmetic doctor or a dermatologist because they could leave a scar, and a professional will know how to make the scar as discreet as possible.

☆ *Tip*

☆ Try to avoid freezing. It often leaves a pale patch.

Cost: Expect to pay £100–£150 per session.
Patient pain rating: 3 (1–10, 1=pain-free)
Treatment time: 15 minutes
How long does it last? 12 months. It can be permanent but they could also re-form; often sessions every 1–2 years are needed.

IPL/lasers for unwanted hair

Hair sprouting around your temples can be a real nuisance. I see quite a few women who get this, mostly Asians from their teens onwards, and it seems to be a hereditary trait.

There are the obvious, albeit short-term solutions such as waxing or shaving it off. However, the no-surgery treatment using lasers and intense pulsed light (IPL) is longer-lasting and very straightforward. Both treatments direct heat energy down the hair shaft into the hair follicle, where it kills the cells responsible for creating the unwanted hair.

Because of the way IPL and laser machines locate the hair by seeking out a difference in colour, they work best on people whose hair colour is much darker than their skin. If there is only a slight difference between skin and hair colour, the machine has to be put on a lower setting and you will need more sessions. Either way, this treatment works well.

Cost: £45–£150 per session depending on treatment area size.
Patient pain rating: 2–3 (1–10, 1=pain-free)
Treatment time: 5–45 minutes, depending on size
How long does it last? Very long-lasting, 2 years or more.

Removing blackheads, whiteheads and milia

Blackheads and whiteheads are grease glands blocked with a mixture of grease and skin. In the case of blackheads there is a bit of pigment (not dirt) in there too. Everyone gets these, but in some people bacteria develop within them, turning them into acne.

Milia look like little white beads. They are little balls made of skin cells that got trapped under the skin instead of getting exfoliated naturally. If you wait long enough they may disappear by themselves, otherwise you can opt for a no-surgery treatment to hasten their departure.

Chemical peels are the clinical exfoliation treatment for blackheads, whiteheads and milia. They exfoliate much more deeply than you are able to with home products. Peels remove the skin that covers the blackheads, whiteheads or milia and squeeze out the contents. Milia can also be pricked out with a (sterile) needle or treated with a laser, which takes off the top of the milia, allowing the contents to be removed.

☆ *Tips*

☆ You can de-clog grease and sweat glands yourself by removing the dead skin that covers them using a loofah or a mild fruit or salicylic acid exfoliant – look out for this on the label, or ask the chemist.

☆ Don't loofah over any inflamed or sore spots. If you scrub at these, you might give yourself scars.

☆ Avoid heavy creams which can cause milia.

☆ See the chapter on Cheeks for more tips and information on spots and acne.

Cost: Expect to pay £100 per session.

Patient pain rating: 2 (1–10, 1=pain-free)

Treatment time: 10 minutes

How long does it last? Permanently, but new ones can develop so you may need maintenance sessions.

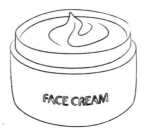

Fatty growths & cysts

Cysts are common on the forehead. Lipomas, although more common on the body, can also develop on the forehead – when they do we remove them using the same technique that we use for cysts.

Lipomas are fatty lumps, roughly two centimetres across, that appear on the forehead (and occasionally other areas) as small bulges underneath the skin that move when you poke them. They don't hurt and they are not dangerous; they just don't look very nice. They seem to run in families, but other than this we don't know what causes them. They usually need to be cut out, and then it is down to how small you can make the scar. So you need to find a plastic surgeon or a doctor with enough expertise who has removed a lot of facial lumps and bumps before.

Fatty (sebaceous) cysts are a very common cosmetic problem. They appear on the forehead as lumps about a centimetre wide. The way to get rid of them is to cut them out. It usually needs three to four stitches, but this is a relatively minor procedure. Your GP will do it, or you can go to a surgeon or a dermatologist.

No-Surgery Treatments for the Chin

The chin is not an area that springs to everyone's mind when we are talking about cosmetic improvements or signs of ageing, but let's not neglect it. A rosy, wrinkly, hairy or saggy chin can be the thing that spoils the look for some. We have corrective no-surgery treatments for these, and occasionally, when people don't like the shape we can enhance it with filler, usually in combination with the cheeks (see also the chapter on Cheeks).

Common problems

- ☆ the chin wrinkle
- ☆ the bobbly chin
- ☆ double chin
- ☆ jowls
- ☆ marionette lines
- ☆ blood vessels (see also the chapter on Cheeks)
- ☆ hairy chin (see also the chapter on Noses)

Filling in the chin wrinkle

This is the downturned-crescent wrinkle that develops just above the chin where the chin muscles are attached. It develops with age, but not on everyone; it depends on your genes and on the shape of your face. It is easy to fill this in with some hyaluronic acid filler and get a good result, but don't forget to massage three times a day for a week post-treatment, to avoid unevenness.

Cost: £200–£350 per session, depending on the depth and length of line.

Patient pain rating: 3–4 (1–10, 1=pain-free)

Treatment time: 15 minutes

How long does it last? 6–9 months

Botox for bobbly chins

This is brought on by a tendency (usually inherited) to subconsciously pucker your chin a lot – when you talk, in your sleep or when you make a serious expression – so that the little dents and mounds become permanent. If you think you do this, try and get out of the habit, but if you can't manage to stop then botox can give you a bit of assistance by making it harder to crumple your chin. If you think your chin has already gone bobbly it is possible to combine botox with a bit of filler to smooth it out. These no-surgery treatments are the only option for this phenomenon; there isn't a surgical alternative.

 Tip

☆ This a job for an experienced practitioner only – one who knows exactly where to put the botox in order to freeze the right muscles. You don't want to end up trading in a bobbly chin for a dribbly one.

Cost: Expect to pay £250 per session.
Patient pain rating: 2– 3 (1– 10, 1=pain-free)
Treatment time: 5 minutes
How long does it last? 3–4 months

Reducing a double chin with radiofrequency remodelling

Small areas of persistent fat around the chin can be a problem from the age of 20 if it is genetic, but this develops more commonly as we age or put on weight. Radiofrequency can actually disperse the fat and tighten the skin to a degree. Don't expect miracles, but you will be pleased. The fat-reducing capabilities of radiofrequency are still being fine-tuned, but I have already seen good results.

Cost: Expect to pay around £300 per session – you may need up to 4 sessions four weeks apart.

Patient pain rating: 4–5. There is a hot sensation at the time of treatment, and red skin that lasts 1–2 hours. (1–10, 1=pain-free)

Treatment time: 10 minutes for each side

How long does it last? Not yet known for sure, but can reasonably expect up to two years.

Reducing jowls with radiofrequency remodelling

Jowls are the bits of our cheeks that descend below the jaw line into little saggy bulges hanging either side of our chin. They start to show in our forties or fifties, and there is not really any preventative action we can take. Some people swear by facial exercises, but I'm doubtful: surely, in the long term, all that exercising and grimacing gives you more stretching and wrinkles.

Skin tightening using radiofrequency remodelling is the no-surgery treatment for jowls. It contracts the skin that has stretched and drooped, giving it a lift, thereby reducing the size of the jowls. Most people see an immediate difference when they look in the mirror after this treatment, and it carries on improving for up to six months. Redefining the jaw line knocks years off a face, so if jowls are a problem for you, tune in and tighten up!

Cost: Expect to pay around £250–£500 per session – you may need up to 4 sessions four weeks apart.
Patient pain rating 4–5 post-treatment. You feel a hot sensation during treatment. (1–10, 1=pain-free)
Treatment time: 10 minutes for each side
How long does it last? Not yet known for sure, but can reasonably expect up to two years.

Lasers for blood vessels

Blood vessels on the chin are common in people with rosacea, but you can also inherit a tendency for them. They can be 'zapped' with a blood-vessel laser or IPL. If you have only got them on your chin, this is a quick treatment and the effects last for a couple of years, as long as you look after and protect your skin.

Cost: Expect to pay £150–£200 per session.
Patient pain rating: 2–3 (1–10, 1=pain-free)
Treatment time: 10 minutes
How long does it last? Permanently, but new ones may develop.

Filling in marionette lines

These are a continuation of nose-to-lip lines. They make people look sad, like the corner of the lip is turned down. There are no home remedies for these other than to stand on your head, take a photo and turn it upside down! However, they can be sorted out with a bit of hyaluronic acid filler, and it works very well. Patients tell me their friends all comment on how well they look.

Cost: Expect to pay £200–£350 per session.
Patient pain rating: 3–4 (1–10, 1=pain-free)
Treatment time: 15 minutes
How long does it last? 6–9 months

On 'the mask of pregnancy' (melasma)

Women can get this when they are pregnant, receiving HRT or taking the contraceptive pill, but sometimes there is no obvious reason. What looks like brown stains appear along the jaw line and across the top lip, cheeks and forehead. This condition seems to be linked to a combination of hormonal change and sun. In most cases it eventually goes away by itself, but for 20 per cent of sufferers it refuses to budge.

This staining can be reduced by up to 50 per cent (sometimes more) with a combination of obsessive sun protection, prescription-strength lightening agents (from a cosmetic doctor) and a course of glycolic peels at the clinic. The chemical peel bleaches and removes the pigment from the surface layers of skin, and the lightening agent slows down the production of more pigment in the deeper layers.

However, for the 20 per cent who are resistant to these treatments, the first bit of sun exposure they get will bring it back. If this is you, don't be downhearted. Medical-research scientists love a challenge, so it shouldn't be long before a no-surgery treatment for resistant melasma comes along. A new type of laser known as a pepper-pot laser looks very promising, but it is still undergoing trials.

Lasers for chin hair

For some as yet unknown reason the chin is the most resistant area to IPL, which means it takes more sessions to get rid of the hairs. The chin is usually prone to spots too, so it might be because chins are more susceptible to hormones. I recommend lasers for these particular hairs as lasers seem to be the most effective way of getting rid of them – more effective than IPL – probably because lasers can penetrate a bit further into the skin. Try and organize the first three treatments a month apart. After that, treatments for any regrowth can be spaced a couple of months apart or more. The top lip and chin are usually treated in one session.

Cost: Expect to pay £75 per session, for 6 or more sessions.

Patient pain rating: 2–3 (1–10, 1=pain-free)

Treatment time: 5 minutes

How long does it last? Once the hair has stopped growing back, it is long-lasting.

No-Surgery Treatments
for the *Neck*

The thickness of your skin varies all over your body. On your neck it is particularly thin, making it less elastic and more fragile. And thin skin is more susceptible to sun damage, stretching and creasing, which is why our necks give away our age. Because the skin is less robust, we can't use any of the more invasive no-surgery treatments that require the skin to repair itself. If we did, it might not heal well, which would leave you with a scar. So we have to stick to gentle treatments for the neck.

Common problems

- ☆ necklace lines
- ☆ neck bands
- ☆ a turkey neck
- ☆ red perfume marks
- ☆ skin tags

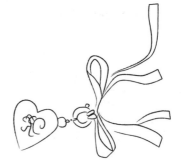

Botox for necklace lines

These are the horizontal creases we make when we bend
our necks forward. By the time we are in our forties or
fifties we have usually developed at least two or three
permanent necklace lines. The only option is botox, which
can soften these slightly. Fillers don't look good because
the skin is so thin they show through and look lumpy.
And don't let anyone try laser-resurfacing your neck,
because the skin is so thin that this will leave you with
scarring. The surgical alternative is a neck lift, but even
surgery isn't great at smoothing out these necklace creases.
It is better for tightening loose skin.

Cost: Expect to pay £200 per session.
Patient pain rating: 2–3 (1–10, 1=pain-free)
Treatment time: 10 minutes
How long does it last? A slight improvement for 3–4 months.

Botox for neck bands

Vertical neck bands are little ridges that eventually fan out from under your chin down towards your collarbones. How much they show varies between individuals. You can see them in the mirror if you tense your neck while gritting your teeth and sticking your chin out. What you see is a very thin muscle just under the skin. As we age, some parts of the muscle form themselves into bands. We don't know why. We can make them less obvious by putting botox directly into the bands to relax them. It doesn't make them go away completely, but it does make them less noticeable. Even a surgical neck-lift, to flatten them by tightening them, would reduce rather than remove them, so botox is not a bad option here.

Cost: Expect to pay £200 per session.
Patient pain rating: 2–3 (1–10, 1=pain-free)
Treatment time: 10 minutes
How long does it last? A good improvement for 3–4 months.

IPL for 'perfume marks'

Some women, usually in their forties upwards, get reddish-brown marks on their necks that run from their ears downwards on both sides. Because this only happens to women and it never happens underneath the neck, the medical profession has come to the conclusion that it is a combination of perfume and sun that causes them. You will really impress your doctor if you use the official name for these: it is Poikiloderma de Cervatte (after the French doctor who first identified and defined the condition). Treating these with IPL can give you a 50–60 per cent improvement.

 Tips

☆ The best treatment is a preventative one: don't forget to cover this area with sun protection; it often gets left out.

☆ Don't perfume your neck, put it on your clothes. If it damages these you can change them.

☆ Remember to schedule your IPL or laser treatments for when you won't have a suntan.

Cost: £250–£300 per session. 2–3 sessions over a 6-month period.

Patient pain rating: 4–5 (1–10, 1=pain-free)

Treatment time: 30 minutes

How long does it last? Long-lasting, unless you re-expose it to the sun, in which case you might need a maintenance treatment.

Getting rid of skin tags

If you find a funny lump of skin, shaped a bit like a pear drop and attached to you via a small thread, it is probably a skin tag. These are very common and run in families. They start appearing when we are in our thirties or later, usually in areas where you get friction, like under your arms or breasts and on the neck where your collar rubs, but they can also develop on the face.

Some people treat skin tags by tying some cotton tightly around the base and waiting for them to blacken and fall off – not for the faint-hearted! I don't recommend this. You are better off getting your doctor to treat them. Removing skin tags is a very minor treatment for a cosmetic doctor. With a bit of local anaesthetic they can be cut off or cauterized (burned off). And if they are particularly large they get a double assault: the bulk gets nipped off with a scalpel and the base gets cauterized.

Cost: Expect to pay around £100–£200 per session.
Patient pain rating: 2–3 with anaesthetic (1–10, 1=pain-free)
Treatment time: 15–30 minutes per session
How long does it last? Forever, but new ones may develop.

Reducing a turkey neck with radiofrequency remodelling

A turkey neck is mostly loose skin. Because the neck skin is so thin and fragile it loses its elasticity. The worst ones I've ever seen were in Australia, which just goes to show what an impact the sun has on fragile skin.

If yours is a fairly mild case of turkey neck, the skin can be tightened with radiofrequency treatments to get a good result; but if there is too much loose skin you will need a surgical neck-lift to get rid of it.

 Tips

☆ Catch it early if you want to take the no-surgery route.

☆ Use sunscreen on the neck – think of those Australians.

☆ Have realistic expectations about the result. This is a subtle change.

Cost: Expect to pay around £250–£500 per session – you may need up to 4 sessions four weeks apart.

Patient pain rating: 4–5. There is a hot sensation at the time of treatment. (1–10, 1=pain-free)

Treatment time: 15 minutes each side

How long does it last? Not yet known for sure, but expect up to two years.

No-Surgery Treatments for the Chest

This is a common area of complaint for women. Problems arise because the skin here is thin, like the neck, and women often wear tops that expose the V-shape, leaving this area of skin open to attack from those nasty UVA and UVB rays. If you don't look after this area it will give you away, however good your face looks.

Common problems

☆ lines from the breast folds when you sleep
☆ age spots
☆ little blood vessels
☆ crêpey skin
☆ keloid scars

Breast fold lines

A lot of women get a couple of these horizontal lines on the chest. They are the permanent traces of where your skin folds when you lie on your side at night. Regular sessions of microdermabrasion (see also the chapter on Eyes) can gradually thicken the skin a little over time (and this treatment can also fade any sun spots). Chemical peels effectively do the same thing, only peels are more likely to cause scarring and pigment changes. Never have a medium or strong peel in this area, only a superficial peel. Breast folds can also be lifted out with filler, but this usually looks lumpy so I wouldn't recommend it. Some doctors use botox, but I don't understand why, because botox works on muscles and it is not a muscular action that causes them, so any benefit is going to be marginal.

☆ *Tip*

☆ To reduce lines and wrinkles, try getting into the habit of sleeping on your back. Apart from the breast folds, when you lie on your side you can develop creases where your eye or cheek get pressed into the pillow. And if you have a favourite side that you lie on more, you will end up with a deeper crease on that side.

Smoothing crêpey skin using IPL & microdermabrasion

Crêpey skin is dry, thin skin. Don't forget to apply sunscreen in this area. Use a cream containing vitamin A and glycolic acid – to get a high-enough potency to make a difference you'll need to get this from a cosmetic doctor or dermatologist. Vitamin A and glycolic acid speed up exfoliation and skin growth as long as you religiously apply them according to the instructions given by your therapist (see also the chapter on Lotions and Potions in Part Two for more information). Microdermabrasion and very mild peels help improve the skin quality here too, but I recommend a combination of IPL and microdermabrasion because I think it works the best.

First you have a series of microdermabrasion sessions. This takes off the dry, crêpey top layers, clearing the way for the IPL light to penetrate more effectively. IPL also fades sun spots, and by repeating this treatment regularly you will gradually see a marked improvement in the quality of your skin – a more even skin tone and a slight skin thickening. It involves a programme of treatments, so it is not a quick fix, but there is a trade-off. It is not an invasive method so it doesn't stop your social life.

I usually recommend microdermabrasion followed by one IPL for three sessions, then microdermabrasion maintenance every three months and an IPL every nine to twelve months (depending on the amount of sun exposure).

 Tip

 ☆ Put sun cream on the v-neck area if your clothes leave it exposed. Believe me, it makes a difference. I can tell by the sharp line of demarcation I see between the smooth skin on the top part of the breast that gets covered up, and that of the v-neck area where it gets sun-damaged.

Microdermabrasion

Cost: Expect to pay £250 for a course of 3 treatments.

Patient pain rating: 2–3 (1–10, 1=pain-free)

Treatment time: 30 minutes

How long does it last? Requires regular maintenance.

IPL

Cost: Expect to pay £250 per session for 2–3 sessions.

Patient pain rating: 3–4 (1–10, 1=pain-free)

Treatment time: 15 minutes

How long does it last? Requires regular maintenance.

IPL, sun spots & blood vessels

The best treatment for fading sun spots on this delicate area is IPL, because it is gentle on the skin's surface (see also the chapter on Anywhere). More aggressive treatments like lasers can give you a scar in the form of a white mark that won't tan, so it looks more obvious than the sun spots did. Don't let your doctor freeze age spots off the chest either, because this leaves white scarring too.

I often treat any broken veins as part of a sun-spot treatment for the chest, because patients commonly have both. It just means going over the blood vessels separately, using a slightly different technique, although sun spots and broken veins can be treated separately, if that is what is required.

Cost: Expect to pay £250 per session for 2–3 sessions.
Patient pain rating: 3–4 (1–10, 1=pain-free)
Treatment time: 15 minutes
How long does it last? Lasts 1–2 years but will slowly recur with more sun exposure.

Keloid scars

These occur on certain parts of the body that tend (for reasons unknown) to produce more scar tissue – the area from the bottom of the ribs upwards, especially between and under the breasts and in the vaccination area of the arm. When the skin gets damaged by something like a picked spot or a breast biopsy, instead of getting a normal scar you get one that continues to grow, up to a couple of centimetres across, and which looks lumpy. If you are Afro-Caribbean you are more likely to get these.

These are tricky to treat. If you cut them out, the lumpy scar grows back again. So instead we work on flattening them and reducing the redness, to make them less noticeable. We flatten them out using steroid injections followed by a period of three months wearing silicone gel patches. Then, once we have done as much flattening as we can, we use a laser to take out the redness.

Cost: Expect to pay £200–£500 for 2–3 injections plus 1–2 sessions with a laser, depending on how many you have.

Patient pain rating: 2–3 (1–10, 1=pain-free)

Treatment t me: 15 minutes

How long does it last? Long-lasting but can recur, in which case you should start steroid injections and silicone patches again as soon as possible, before they grow any bigger.

No-Surgery Treatments
for Hands
and Underarms

Look, Doctor, my bones are showing!
I can see the blood vessels and the skin looks all crêpey.

If you want to gauge a person's age you look at the backs of their hands and their neck. Hands are subjected to more wear and tear, and people often forget to put sun cream on them. The thing people dislike most is sun spots, also referred to on hands as 'liver spots' or 'age spots'. The French name for sun spots translates into English as 'cemetery medallions' – and if that doesn't jolt you into looking after your hands, then nothing will.

The second most common complaint is crêpey skin that wrinkles when you put your hand flat. The skin on our hands thins by 60–70 per cent over 40–50 years so your bones and veins start to show through it – which is another thing my patients don't like.

We also treat women and men for excess sweating on hands and underarms. It can be a socially debilitating condition, making this a life-changing treatment for some. Which could also be said of the treatment for long-term underarm hair removal – this can save you hours that you would otherwise while away engaged in awkward postures in the bathroom.

Common hand problems

☆ liver spots/age spots/sun spots on hands (most common)

☆ thin, crêpey skin

☆ too veiny

☆ too bony

☆ excessive sweating

Removing highly visible blue veins

These are the blue motorways-on-a-map veins you can see through the back of the hand, which get more noticeable over time as the skin there gets thinner. Some surgeons cut them out, but this leads to problems – people have ended up with a network of little blood vessels that look like a bruise. In my opinion, more obvious veins are good – if you collapse and need an operation, it is easier for the anaesthetist to see where to put the drip in!

Loss of fat between bones

It is very difficult to do anything about this. Fat can be transferred from the tummy or buttock to the hand, via injections. This wouldn't require a general anaesthetic but this is not on the no-surgery treatment menu so it is best left to surgeons. The results I've seen are not good – it either leaves the hands looking lumpy or they don't look any different from before.

Common underarm problems

☆ skin tags (see also the chapter on the Neck)
☆ excess sweating
☆ hair
☆ batwings

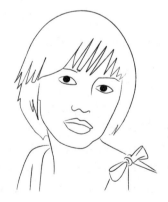

IPL for fading sun spots

IPL is the treatment of choice; it works really nicely. You should see a 60–70 per cent improvement that will last, provided you keep your hands out of the sun as much as possible, wear a sunscreen and go for yearly maintenance sessions.

Sun spots can also be removed using pigment lasers that take out the brown colour, but the downside of this route is that it leaves you with a white mark instead. The white mark won't tan and looks obvious on darker skins. Similarly, individual sun spots can be laser-resurfaced off, but, again, this leaves a white mark behind. So I prefer the IPL method.

 Tips

☆ Don't let anyone laser-resurface the whole back of your hand – the skin is too thin. It could leave permanent white scars.

☆ Use a handcream containing sunscreen and vitamin A, and reapply it regularly.

Cost: £250 per session. You'll need 2 or 3 sessions 3 months apart and then yearly maintenance sessions.

Patient pain rating: 3–4 (1–10, 1=pain-free)

Treatment time: 15 minutes for both hands

How long does it last? For as long as you protect your hands from the sun and continue with yearly maintenance sessions.

Plumping up thin, crêpey skin

Peeling treatments, microdermabrasion and red light all
help to plump the skin. You can combine two of them, or all
three. Microdermabrasion followed by red light is a good
combination: usually three to six of each, depending on
how quickly your skin responds. You can get a 50 per cent
improvement if you have a course of one a month for six
months, which you can then maintain with a top-up
treatment every three to six months.

 Tips

☆ Ask your practitioner to do your hands while he does your
  face – it will cost less.

☆ Get some cream containing vitamin A and glycolic acid from
  your cosmetic doctor. Vitamin A and glycolic acid speed up
  exfoliation and skin growth.

Cost: £75– £100 per session for any one of these treatments.

Patient pain rating: 1 (1– 10, 1=pain-free)

Treatment time: 15 minutes (both hands) for any one of these
treatments.

How long does it last? There should be a 50 per cent
improvement.

Botox for hand-sweating

Excess sweating can be a real social problem for people, which botox can resolve because injecting it into the sweat glands effectively switches them off for up to six months. When I was in training for this, the first girl that turned up didn't want to shake hands. She said she couldn't read books or touch paper because it left a handprint and her social contact was limited: she was worried people would think she was dirty. The treatment involves first injecting a local anaesthetic in the wrist – and as hands are extra-sensitive, injections can be quite uncomfortable here – but the girl refused the anaesthetic. I watched my mentor give her 40 or 50 botox injections in the skin of one hand while she sat quite still. 'This transforms my life,' she said. 'I am ready for the pain.'

We usually give the patient some anaesthetic cream and a plastic glove which makes the cream absorb better. After the treatment, the hands feel odd for 24 hours or so. The botox starts to work within a couple of weeks.

Cost: Expect to pay £500 per session.
Patient pain rating: 4–5 with anaesthetic cream (1–10, 1=pain-free)
Treatment time: 30 minutes
How long does it last? Up to 6 months.

Botox for underarm sweating

We do this treatment for men and women. It takes between
25 and 30 tiny superficial botox injections in each armpit. It
doesn't need an anaesthetic as injections in the armpit are
relatively painless.

Before we give botox treatments for excess sweating on the
hands or under the arms we do the sweat-gland-detector
trick, to determine where we need to put the injections.
It is also a way of making sure the problem is down to 'real'
excess sweating, and not 'imagined' excess sweating. We
paint iodine onto the skin, then sprinkle starch on top. Little
dark dots appear because the salt in the sweat turns the
iodine black. These dots show us where to inject the botox.

 Tips

☆ You can buy over-the-counter products that contain
   aluminium hydroxide. Some of my patients say these help a
   bit. If these products were really good I doubt these patients
   would come to see me, but you might want to give them a try.

☆ Surgery, although permanent, is not a good option for under
   the armpits. It leaves a scar and it can lead to nerve problems
   or permanent pins and needles.

Cost: Expect to pay £500 – £600 per session.

Patient pain rating: 3–4 (1–10, 1=pain-free)

Treatment time: 15 minutes

How long does it last? 5–6 months

Removing hair using IPL

This is the most successful area for hair removal as the underarm responds well to IPL. It takes three to four sessions, a month apart, but you get a good result – the hairs generally don't grow back. Lasers work just as effectively, but because the IPL machine treats a larger area with each 'zap', the laser treatment may take slightly longer.

☆ *Tip:*

☆ Don't tell your doctor that you are bothered by wrinkles in your armpit – she will think you are mad!

Cost: Expect to pay £250 for 3 sessions.

Patient pain rating: 2– 3 (1– 10, 1=pain-free)

Treatment time: 15 minutes

How long does it last? Two years or more.

Reducing batwings with radiofrequency remodelling

Batwings is the pet name for the skin on the under part of the arm that, as we get older, becomes loose, holds fat and hangs down in a rather unpleasant way, then flaps about when you shake your hands. Radiofrequency does two things here. It tightens the skin and reduces the fat. At my clinic we can change the setting on our system to switch between these two functions. Expect a 25 per cent improvement overall.

The surgical option is liposuction, but this only works when you have got good skin tone that will tighten itself up once you have had the fat removed.

Cost: £200–£300 per session for both arms – 6–8 sessions probably needed, 1–2 weeks apart.

Patient pain rating: 4–5. A hot sensation at time of treatment. Red skin that lasts 1–2 hours. (1–10, 1=pain-free)

Treatment time: 10 minutes each side

How long does it last? Not yet known for sure, but expect up to two years.

No-Surgery Treatments for the Trunk, Front and Back

Around the waist it is usually the shape and texture people are not happy with: lumpy bits, love handles, stomach rolls and cellulite. There are no-surgery treatments for shrinking stubborn bits of flab that don't seem to shift, even with dieting. This can happen at any age. These treatments can help with contouring but not weight loss; they are not an alternative to dieting, so you need to have realistic expectations.

We can also tidy up unwanted moles, hair, sun spots, plus a few little nuisances that are unique to this area. Then there is the dreaded stretch mark: though cosmetic science hasn't developed a method of removing these completely – yet – we can make them less obvious.

Common problems

☆ shape
☆ little red dots (Campbell de Morgan Spots)
☆ raised brown spots (seborrhoeic keratoses)
☆ hair
☆ stretch marks
☆ sun spots/sun damage on shoulder
☆ little blood vessels – small blue/red vessels mostly on the lower chest and tummy

Sun spots and sun damage

Sun spots gather across shoulders that have seen a lot of sun, making the skin look mottled and aged, but there are no-surgery treatments for fading them (see the chapter on Anywhere for details). Once they have been faded, and provided you keep them out of the sun, you can dig out your favourite little backless number and show them off.

Endermology for cellulite

Regular endermology treatments can effect a minor change to shape and reduce cellulite. The effects are gradual and it works best on younger patients, whose cellulite tends to show mostly when they move. Endermology is not suitable for anyone who is overweight, or for more mature women whose cellulite is well established; that is, fixed and still visible when the muscles are fully relaxed.

Cost: £550 for 14 sessions. You will need 2–3 sessions per week for 5 weeks and then maintenance every 3 months to get a result.

Patient pain rating: 1–2 (1–10, 1=pain-free)

Treatment time: 45 minutes per session

How long does it last? 3-monthly maintenance sessions will be necessary for a sustained effect.

Removing little red tummy spots using gentle lasers

I see quite a few patients with a rash of tiny cherry-red dots on the front of their tummies. Each spot is roughly a millimetre wide and can be either flat or raised. They are called Campbell de Morgan Spots after the gentleman who first identified them and they are not cancerous, just a bit unsightly.

These commonly appear in men or women of 40 plus, on the trunk of the body, for reasons unknown. They are easily treated with a blood-vessel laser. One zap is all it takes. The spots instantly turn from deep red to grey, and then in a few days they shrivel and vanish. I once treated 170 of these on one man. One treatment is usually enough, but people who get them tend to get more.

Cost: Expect to pay £200 per session.
Patient pain rating: 2–3 (1–10, 1=pain-free)
Treatment time: 2–3 seconds per spot
How long does it last? Permanently, but new ones are likely to appear.

Tummy & back spots

Another small irritation with a big name is seborrhoeic keratosis: little brown raised oval warty, scaly lumps, about a centimetre across, that appear on the tummy and back. They are not malignant, just a nuisance, and they are easy to remove. We can scrape them off with a scalpel, freeze them off, or remove them with a laser. All methods require a local anaesthetic and all leave a pale scar. At first the area looks bright pink, but this gradually fades to pale pink, and eventually turns paler than the skin around it. Once removed they don't come back, but you could get new ones.

 Tips

☆ These grow bigger over time. The sooner you get them removed, the smaller the pale scar will be.

☆ If you have a lot, get them checked out by your doctor, because, very rarely, they can indicate a more serious disease.

☆ Obviously, don't let any mole get sunburnt.

Cost: £100+ per session, depending on how many you have.
Patient pain rating: 2–3, local anaesthetic (1–10, 1=pain-free)
Treatment time: 15–30 minutes, depending on amount of spots
How long does it last? Permanently

IPL for unwanted hair

We get a lot of male patients who don't like the hair on their back, mainly across the shoulders, but in Mediterranean men it can be on the lower back as well. Also, but more rarely, women have this treatment for excessive pubic hair, or the triangle of hair below the navel, nipple hair and around the bikini line.

There is always the option of waxing it, like the Premiership football players (why do they do this?), but in the no-surgery clinic it can be removed using IPL or lasers. However, the high testosterone in men drives and strengthens the hair follicle, so the hair tends to grow back, which means hair removal on men is more of a maintenance process involving six-monthly treatments – not ideal, but it lasts longer than a wax. This is particularly popular with gay men and with men whose wives don't like their hairy backs.

☆ *Tips*

☆ Do not go for IPL treatments when you are tanned because the machine finds the hair by hunting out the darker colour, so this will confuse it and burn your skin.

☆ Do not pluck or bleach the hair before you go for laser treatment, because the laser won't be able to find the hair, so it won't destroy it.

☆ Neither IPL nor lasers can get rid of every single hair, so expect a 70–80 per cent improvement – slightly less for men.

☆ Any hair that grows back tends to be finer and a lighter colour, in women and in men.

Cost: Expect to pay £1,000 for 6–8 sessions – quite pricey, but the effects are very long-lasting.

Patient pain rating: 2–3 for women. 4–5 for men. It is always more for men! (1–10, 1=pain-free)

Treatment time: 30–45 minutes

How long does it last? Can be permanent, mostly is long-lasting.

Retin-A & lasers for fast-fading stretch marks

Stretch marks are scars in the skin where the skin has lost its elasticity, like an elastic band that has lost its ping. People have a genetic predisposition for these, which is set off by rapid weight gain, or by steroid treatments for medical problems.

This treatment is good for women who have had a baby and are going on holiday. It makes stretch marks less obvious by quickly fading the red-mauve marks to a paler silvery grey, which would otherwise happen naturally over 12 months. With laser treatment it takes only two weeks, and with Retin-A it takes between four and six weeks, but Retin-A is cheaper than laser treatment.

Once the stretch marks have turned grey and silvery, there is nothing further we can do – nothing yet, anyway, but I am hopeful that there will be in future.

Tips

☆ Don't get too excited about any new treatments for stretch
   marks. Wait until they have been thoroughly tested.

☆ All you can do to try to prevent stretch marks is to keep the
   skin moist with oil or moisturizer. Don't invest in a specific
   product, just use a good, plain moisturizer.

☆ Don't use Retin-A or any other products containing vitamin A
   while you are pregnant, but you can as soon as the baby is born.

Retin-A

Cost: Expect to pay £50 per 60g tube of Retin-A.

Patient pain rating: 1 (1– 10, 1=pain-free)

Treatment time: Takes 4– 6 weeks for marks to go grey.

How long does it last? Permanently

Lasers

Cost: Expect to pay £250 per session.

Patient pain rating: 3 (1– 10, 1=pain-free)

Treatment time: 15 minutes, and they take two weeks to go grey.

How long does it last? Permanently

Radiofrequency remodelling for waist-line bulges

Radiofrequency waves can travel through the skin without damaging it to achieve two things: tighten it up and reduce fat and cellulite. Remember, this is a new treatment. We don't have scientific studies yet, though these are in the pipeline, but we do have lots of anecdotal evidence from France and the US where radiofrequency has been used to reduce bulgy bits for a couple of years already.

You should see an improvement within 2–3 sessions, but you may need 6–8 treatments at weekly intervals to reach optimum reduction. It is only suitable for persistent areas of fat, and is not a treatment for obesity. It works best in younger age groups. The surgical alternative is liposuction and a tummy tuck.

Cost: Expect to pay £300 per session. You will probably need up to 6–8 sessions, 1– 2 weeks apart.

Patient pain rating: 2–3 (1–10, 1=pain-free)

Treatment time: 30 minutes

How long does it last? Provided you don't put on weight, this treatment is long-lasting. It should stay the same for at least two years or longer.

No-Surgery Treatments for Legs

Those first clement days of spring signal that summer is not far off and legs will soon be uncovered. This usually prompts a surge of requests for vein treatments from ladies in their thirties and above, particularly women whose jobs involve standing around or sitting in the same position for most of the day, which can build up enough pressure in the blood vessels of the legs to cause a blowout.

Pregnancy also ups the pressure in the leg veins, because the baby squishes your blood vessels, especially if you lie on your back. So it is better for your legs if you sleep on your side when you are pregnant.

We Brits spend more time and money on beauty treatments for our faces than the rest of our bodies. In sunnier climes women are more conscious of how the rest of their body looks because it is more often on view. In Italy and Spain, cellulite is actually recognized as a medical condition and treatments for reducing it are widely used, whereas in the UK women generally start to worry about their cellulite the week before their summer holidays.

Common problems

☆ veins
☆ cellulite
☆ hair

Removing visible veins with microsclerotherapy

There are different types of visible leg veins, and this is the treatment for removing the tiny little blue or red ones that look like biro marks on the outer or inner surface of the thigh or calf. It is not for varicose veins, which are bigger, curly, lumpy blue veins.

Veins are like columns of blood. The lower you go down the column, the higher the pressure. Because the legs are the lowest bits of us, you get the odd blood vessel that can't take the strain. A tiny, tiny blood vessel, which you normally wouldn't see, balloons to a visible size and pops out onto the surface of the skin.

If you get a lot of these you are probably genetically susceptible to them, so take some preventative action: when you are sitting or standing for a long time, keep that blood flowing by regularly changing your position; and arm yourself with some support tights from the chemist. Don't baulk at this: these days you can get all sorts of styles so they don't look any different from normal tights.

With this treatment a chemical that seals the blood vessel is injected into each tiny vein through a very fine needle. In order to get a good result, the doctor or nurse needs polarized light and strong magnification to make it possible to see the chemical entering the vein, otherwise she might miss it and not realize.

147

You can expect a 70 to 80 per cent improvement within six weeks of the treatment, and a bit of bruising, redness or blotchiness for the first two. Side-effects are very rare. In a few cases little brown stains, like pencil marks, can appear, but these fade within a year and are less obvious than the original blood vessel. Patients of mine who have had these say they prefer the faint brown stain to those horribly unsightly veins. Even more unusual is a bit of brown matting: a fine mesh of little blood vessels that looks like a red bruise. It usually goes by itself within three to six months, but if it doesn't you can have it injected or lasered. Extremely rarely a small scar may form, which fades over 6–12 months.

☆ Tips

☆ If this problem recurs soon after treatment it is probably because you have underlying varicose veins. You should sort out the bigger varicose veins before doing the little ones, because the varicose ones can cause the little ones.

☆ Autumn is the ideal time to start this treatment, so that your legs are ready for the following summer. Spring is leaving it a bit late, so plan ahead.

☆ Pick a practitioner who uses magnification and polarized light if you can – they will get a better view of what they are doing.

☆ For two weeks after the treatment you will have to avoid vigorous exercise and anything that will heat up your legs, like sunbathing, saunas or hot baths. We don't want to encourage the blood to circulate through those veins too much.

☆ Lasers don't work well on this area, but as lasers become more technically advanced this is likely to change.

☆ We recommend our patients wear support tights for 1–2 weeks post treatment. The benefits of this are not proven, but it may help to speed up the healing process and it can't do any harm.

Cost: Expect to pay £150–£200 per session. Needs 2–3 sessions with a couple of months between each one.

Patient pain rating: 2–3 (1–10, 1=pain-free)

Treatment time: 30–45 minutes

How long does it last? If you are genetically predisposed to them you will get new ones, in which case you will need treatment every 2–3 years.

Varicose veins

These are big blue vessels that come up on the inner thigh and calf and sometimes hurt or make the skin go blue around your ankle. If they are a family trait you will get them from your twenties onwards. Some doctors or surgeons offer sclerotherapy for these bigger veins, which is the same method as microsclerotherapy but done on a grander scale. However, this doesn't work as well on varicose veins as it does on little veins. You would probably be better off having varicose veins surgically removed. With modern techniques it involves minimal downtime and leaves only tiny scars.

Permanent hair removal

IPL and lasers have revolutionized long-term hair removal. They last much longer than shaving or waxing and can cover areas that would take too long with electrolysis: it would take years to treat one leg with electrolysis and with IPL or lasers you can do a leg in 30 minutes.

Leg hairs have a slower growth cycle than hair on other parts of the body, so you need to spread out the treatments more. To start with you will need two to three sessions with a month in between each one. Then, if any hairs do pop up again you'll need a top-up every two to three months until no more grow back. To get your legs hair-free it is going to take a maximum of six to eight sessions, spread over a year to eighteen months, but it may take fewer sessions if you have fair skin and dark hair, because this makes the IPL and lasers more efficient.

☆ Tips

- ☆ This treatment won't work if you have a tan, so plan ahead.
- ☆ This works best on white legs and black hairs.
- ☆ This doesn't work on black skin.
- ☆ This doesn't work on fair or grey hair.
- ☆ This is more successful on women than men, because testosterone makes the hair follicles more resilient.
- ☆ If it is not working on you, you will know within a couple of sessions.
- ☆ There is no significant difference between lasers and IPL. Both are good.
- ☆ Watch out for any moles appearing on your lower leg. This area gets the most sun exposure because it remains uncovered when you are wearing shorts and skirts. I see a lot of skin cancers developing here.

Cost: Expect to pay £150 per session for just the lower legs, £250 per session for full legs.

Patient pain rating: 2–3 (1–10, 1=pain-free)

Treatment time: 45 mins

How long does it last? After a course of 6–8 treatments, hopefully permanently.

Reducing cellulite with endermology

Cellulite develops on thighs and buttocks. The present theory is that it is a circulatory problem. Slow blood flow leads to a build-up of toxins, water and retention of fat. This makes the fat cells bulge, which is what causes the dimpling in the skin.

Imagine the surface of a honeycomb – the holes are fat cells but there is too much of a build-up of fat and it bulges out of the cell, causing the structure to become ridged and scarred. In women it bulges out, but in men it bulges downwards, and this is something to do with oestrogen. The endermology tactic is to break down the scarred honeycomb cells so the fat can escape. However, how this treatment works is theoretical; nothing has been proved to date.

There are several stages to the development of cellulite. At first, it only shows when you contract your muscles. If it becomes established, it is visible when the victim is sitting or lying down. If you are in the early stages these treatments can prevent cellulite getting worse. This doesn't seem to work in women in their fifties onwards because that scarring becomes harder to break down. I would recommend it for younger people with mild cellulite, because it does seem to work if you keep up the treatments and eat and exercise well.

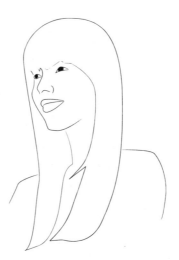

☆ *Tip*

☆ Endermology isn't suitable for anyone who is overweight, as it targets skin fat not body fat.

Cost: Expect to pay £600 for a course of 2 treatments per week for 7 weeks, and £70 per session for top-up treatments.

Patient pain rating: 1–2 (1–10, 1=pain-free)

Treatment time: 45 minutes

How long does it last? You will need maintenance sessions every 3 months to maintain the benefits.

Myth: Coffee or salt can cause cellulite.

There is no proof that any particular food is linked to cellulite. However, the diet that is best for your skin is a balanced one.

Myth: Having cellulite means dieting.

This is false: although we can't explain exactly why cellulite occurs, we know it is not just about weight.

Myth: If you have cellulite it means you need to lose weight.

☆ Tips

☆ Anything that increases the circulation might help: diet and exercise and mechanical treatments.

☆ There are lots of creams and lotions advertised for the treatment of cellulite. Don't waste your money because nothing has been proven and when you understand the structure – the ridged, hard, honeycomb structure – you can understand that a cream can't do much.

☆ I see girls on the underground anxiously slugging water because they think you can't get enough. It is like mineral water has become a fashion accessory. Free up your handbags – there is no need to drink more than 1.5 litres a day, unless you have been advised to for medical reasons.

☆ Liposuction does not treat cellulite. The cellulite is fat that is attached to the skin. Liposuction can only remove fat that is underneath the skin. If a surgeon started tackling cellulite with liposuction, the machine could cause serious damage.

☆ There is a load of machinery coming on to the market combining lasers and light treatments to tackle cellulite, but whether they work has yet to be proven.

Reducing flab & cellulite

Some radiofrequency machines have a special setting that increases the frequency of the waves by 30 to 40 per cent, sending the pulses deeper into the skin where it can reach the cellulite. The waves break down the little honeycomb compartments and disperse the fat inside them. It also reduces the fat, to the extent that you can measure the difference before and after the treatment. This usually gets a high patient satisfaction rating after six to eight sessions, particularly in women aged between 20 and 40.

Cost: Expect to pay around £300 per session – you may need up to 6–8 in sessions, 1–2 weeks apart.

Patient pain rating: 4–5. You feel a hot sensation during treatment. (1–10, 1=pain-free)

Treatment time: 10 minutes each side

How long does it last? Not yet known for sure, but expect up to two years.

No-Surgery Treatments for *Anywhere*

There are some problems that can pop up just about anywhere on the face and body.

Common problems

☆ tattoos

☆ sun spots

☆ removing moles, lumps, bumps and warts

☆ unwanted hair

☆ birthmarks

☆ scars (see also the chapter on Cheeks)

Colour lasers for tattoos

Removing tattoos isn't a straightforward job. It takes two types of laser to remove all the colours, and the approach varies depending on the type of tattoo you have. Green, yellow and purple are harder to remove than black or red, and highly professional tattoos are harder to remove because they are deeper in the skin. Poor-quality tattoos are often made with cheap ink containing impurities that react to the laser by changing colour, often to dark black. If this happens it becomes a two-stage process because you need to be lasered again to remove the black.

The heat from the tattoo laser shatters the pigment and the immune system clears away the remnants. This treatment typically takes 10–15 sessions and is quite painful, although you can use an anaesthetic cream.

 Tips

☆ Make sure you have a test first to check for strange reactions to impurities in the pigment.

☆ It is important to see someone who removes tattoos regularly because it takes know-how to do a good job.

☆ Don't let anyone cut them out or inject them with chemicals, because this will leave you with scars.

☆ If your tattoo contains colours other than black and red, you need to go to a clinic with two types of laser to have all the colours removed.

Cost: Depends on tattoo size and what colours you have in it.
Patient pain rating: 2– 5 (1– 10, 1=pain-free)
Treatment time: Up to 30 mins depending on tattoo size.
How long does it last? Permanently

IPL for fading sun spots

Sun spots look like freckles because they are small, flat and brown, but unlike freckles they don't develop naturally. A sun spot is formed by pigment cells grouping together in response to sunlight, which starts to happen from your late teens onwards. So you get them on your hands, the top of your cheeks, your forehead, your shoulders, and around the v-neck area of your chest – all areas that are frequently exposed.

I think IPL is the best no-surgery treatment for sun spots. Immediately after the treatment the sun spots look darker, but within one to two weeks they flake and fade. After two or three treatments they will be much paler, although eventually they will darken again, so you need to repeat this treatment every couple of years.

 Tip

☆ Stay in the shade, use a sunscreen and your sun spots will fade – not completely, but they will be much less noticeable. You can also buy lightening creams from the chemist or clinic that slow down your pigment production.

Cost: Expect to pay around £200 per session.
Patient pain rating: 4–5 (1–10, 1=pain-free)
Treatment time: 5 minutes per hand
How long does it last? Effects last 6–18 months.

Strong lasers for sun spots

Extra-large, dark sun spots can be removed by laser. Once removed, no trace of sun spot remains except a pale mark only noticeable on darker skin, so this only works on fair skins. Each time the laser is passed across the sun spot it removes very tiny amounts of skin, until all the pigment has gone. You can have a local anaesthetic or cream to make it feel more comfortable.

Cost: Expect to pay around £200–£300 per session.
Patient pain rating: 4–5 (1–10, 1=pain-free)
Treatment time: 10 minutes per session
How long does it last? Permanently

Pigment lasers for sun spots

Again, this removes the sun spot but replaces it with a pale mark that would show up on darker skins. Compared to strong lasers, this will probably heal quicker, but the results are much the same.

Cost: Expect to pay £100–£200 per session.
Patient pain rating: 5–6 (1–10, 1=pain-free)
Treatment time: 15 minutes
How long does it last? Forever, but other sun spots may appear.

☆ *Tip*

☆ Freezing, cauterizing and cutting out sun spots leaves scars or white marks that might be worse than the original spot, so I don't recommend these methods.

Moles, lumps, bumps & warts

There are so many different types of lumps and bumps: brown moles, hairy moles, viral warts … and a load of benign things that can all be chopped or cauterized. However, there are also lots that are not straightforward, so whatever it is, show it to your GP or skin specialist first, to rule out anything dangerous. If they say it is nothing to worry about they won't be able to remove it on the NHS. If you want it removed for cosmetic reasons, this is something a cosmetic doctor, dermatologist or plastic surgeon can do.

There are various ways of removing things: shaving off (with a scalpel), cutting out, lasering off, freezing or cauterizing. The method used depends on the position and size of the bump. Cauterizing works best on smaller things like warts and skin tags and it is efficient because it is fast, sterile and heals quickly. Shaving is better than cutting if the bump is in a place where the skin is very tight, making it difficult to bring the edges together for stitching. Stitches involve a bit more maintenance because they have to come out on day five, but if it is a bigger lump that needs fixing, stitches can achieve a neat hairline scar. All of these require a small anaesthetic under and around the lump or bump.

 Tips

☆ Use silicone gel patches for two to three months after surgery to reduce scarring. You can buy them in a chemist.

☆ Don't let anyone cut a mole on an area where the skin is very tight, like the bridge of your nose, because the scar will definitely stretch. In this case the operation should be carried out by a plastic surgeon.

☆ Don't be blinded with science and assume lasers have magical healing powers. When it comes to removing lumps and bumps, lasers are just an alternative way of shaving them off.

☆ Warts may take a couple of sessions to remove. This is normal, and a few will repeatedly come back whatever you do. Warts are caused by a virus, and what often happens is we suddenly develop antibodies to the virus and they vanish. It is as if the immune system wakes up to the fact there is a virus in the skin and reacts. This explains why many old wives' tales for treating warts can appear to be successful.

Cost: £100 for shaving or cauterizing, £200 for cutting and stitches
Patient pain rating: 2–3 (1–10, 1=pain-free)
Treatment time: 15 minutes
How long does it last? Permanently for most of them.

Scar-reducing methods

However the scar came about – injury, previous operation, self-inflicted or acne – the approach is the same: we are aiming to make scars less noticeable and easier to cover with makeup. It is a myth that we can waft scars away with a laser. What we can do is lighten the colour, reduce bumps and lift depressions. We can't erase scars completely.

If your cosmetic doctor achieves a 50 per cent improvement then he or she has done a good job. I say this because I don't want you to be disappointed. Many who come to see me think I can just zap a scar away with a laser, but improvement comes through a combination of treatments which are carried out in stages, usually over a 12-month period. Certain scars are bumps that are relatively easy to flatten using lasers, but most scars are depressions, so they are lower than the surface of the skin around them. For example, acne scars are either soft dents, known as rolling scars, which you can flatten out using your finger and thumb, or deep, dark holes known as ice-pick scars.

☆ Tips

- ☆ Don't pick.
- ☆ Keep the skin moisturized and don't pick.
- ☆ If you have a fresh scar, get some silicone gel squares from your pharmacy. They help the skin heal by excluding the air. We don't understand how it works but the tests show it does, as long as the scar is a new one.
- ☆ Spot creams can reduce inflammation and infection.

Subcision treatment for depression scars

This is a treatment for a depression scar. It is a useful, permanent way of getting some improvement. The scar sinks inwards because it is being pulled down by tendrils of contracted scar tissue. We try and break some of these little tendrils by moving a needle around in a fan-shape motion inside the dip of the scar (with a local anaesthetic).

Flattening depressions by closing or skin grafting

If you have a large ice-pick scar it can be cut out and the edges brought together to leave a flatter fine line, instead of a dark hole. Occasionally, if the ice-pick scar is really big we can take a bit of skin from behind the ear and fill it, but we don't do this often.

Reducing bumpy scars with superficial peels, lasers and microdermabrasion

All three methods effectively do the same thing. That is, they help reduce any ridges or edges and stimulate collagen to help plump up the depressions and make the normal skin healthier.

Removing redness or darker scars using lasers

With blood-vessel lasers you can take out the pinkness so the scar becomes more skin-coloured. Sometimes in darker skin-types the scar goes darker than the surrounding skin, and in other cases it can go paler. We can use lasers to lighten dark patches but we can't darken light ones – you can take the pigment out but you can't put it back in.

Using fillers to raise depressions

This is an alternative if subcision does not work so well. We can use a filler such as Restylane to push the depression up so that it is level with the surrounding skin.

Subcision

Cost: Expect to pay £100 per session. Usually requires 2– 3 sessions.

Patient pain rating: 3– 4 (1– 10, 1=pain-free)

Treatment time: 15 minutes

How long does it last? Permanently

Restylane

Cost: Expect to pay from £200 per session.

Patient pain rating 2– 3 (1– 10, 1=pain-free)

Treatment time: 15– 30 minutes

How long does it last? 9– 12 months

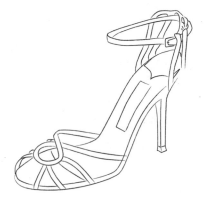

Removing unwanted hair by IPL, laser or electrolysis

If there are less than 10 hairs, electrolysis is a cheaper way to get rid of them and more widely available in beauty salons than IPL and laser treatments. Electrolysis also has the advantage when dealing with grey or blonde hairs because lasers and IPL don't work on light coloured hair. But electrolysis falls short when it comes to larger numbers of hairs because it removes them one hair at a time whereas IPL and lasers can remove many hairs with a single zap.

The most common hair-removal treatments we do for women are the top lip, chin and sideburn area, and the forehead on Asian women. The chin and jawline often need more sessions than other areas because hairs here are more resistant to treatment, and those with darker skins often need more sessions because darker skin requires a lower power setting.

☆ *Tip*

☆ Always have a test patch first.

Cost: Expect to pay £60– £250 per session.

Patient pain rating: 2– 3 (1– 10, 1=pain-free)

Treatment time: Between 10 and 30 minutes depending on the size of area.

How long does it last? Long-lasting once regrowth is treated, unless the area is very resistant to treatment, as in male back hair (see also the chapter on the Trunk).

Lasers for birthmarks

There are two types of birthmark: brown ones and red ones.
The commonest red ones are called port-wine stains and
they are usually positioned on one side of the face. This type
can be treated with lasers.

The brown type of birthmark comes in various shapes and
sizes and in general there is less you can do to remove these.
Nevertheless, it is worth discussing laser and surgery
options with a specialist, as there are some exceptions.

Cost: £200 per session, you may need 1– 15 sessions depending on
the size. Port-wine-stain laser removal is also available on the NHS.

Patient pain rating: 5 using a pulsed dye laser, which is the most
effective, or 3– 4 using IPL (1– 10, 1=pain-free)

Treatment time: Depends on birthmark size; average is 30 min.

How long does it last? Permanent, up to 70 per cent
improvement.

Part 2

The Treatments

- ☆ how they work
- ☆ myths
- ☆ background stories about their usage
- ☆ what it is like to experience them: anecdotes and personal stories
- ☆ side-effects

Botox

How it works

How botox treats wrinkles is something doctors discovered quite by accident almost 20 years ago. When they were using it to treat people with facial tics around the eye area they noticed it also made their wrinkles improve.

If you scrunch up a cotton hanky a few times, you will put creases into it. Your skin creases too, when you scrunch it up with facial expressions. It doesn't happen when we are young because young skin is full of elastic fibres that make it spring back into place. But as we gradually lose this elasticity, our facial expressions leave creases in our skin, which we call wrinkles.

Botox temporarily weakens the muscles that gather your skin into folds, making it crease-proof enough to prevent wrinkles becoming established. Your doctor will pinpoint which muscles to weaken. When injected, botox attaches itself to the target muscle. Once it wears off, usually after four months, the muscles regenerate and regain enough strength to start creasing up your skin again.

Is it safe?

There are literally hundreds of studies showing botox is perfectly safe as long as it is used in the recommended amounts, and we only use tiny amounts to treat wrinkles. But it is a prescription drug, so only doctors are allowed to use it. Even nurses can't give botox injections unless a doctor is present, chiefly because if you are given too much you could spend the next three months with droopy eyelids, eyebrows that don't work together (one goes up while the other goes down), or, if you have too much near your mouth, drooling. Not a good look. There are drops available to help reduce these symptoms, but otherwise it is just a case of waiting for them to settle down. So here is my top tip: Don't get your botox done in a nail salon; go to a qualified, experienced doctor.

You should not have botox if you:

☆ are taking muscle relaxants
☆ have a muscle-weakening disorder
☆ are pregnant
☆ are breastfeeding
☆ have alcohol in your system – the injections are more likely to give you bruises and alcohol can make the botox spread to muscles you don't want to treat.

Side-effects

☆ About 10 per cent of people say they get a headache within 24 hours of having botox injections. We don't know why. It is not necessarily the botox that causes the headache. They usually resolve within 48 hours.

☆ Whenever you pierce or scratch skin enough to make it bleed, there is always a chance of it getting inflamed. Leave your face alone, do not apply makeup for a few hours, and avoid poking around where you have had the injections. After three to four hours you can touch the area and put makeup on it. By then the tiny holes the needles made will have sealed over.

☆ Sometimes the injection can give you a teeny bruise around the needle-prick, which may take a week to disappear but should be easy to conceal with a bit of makeup.

 Tips

☆ If you are having botox for the first time, ask your practitioner to give you the minimum they think you will need, and then, if in a month it hasn't done the trick, a top-up. Your practitioner should agree to this as part of the initial fee because it is a good way to avoid giving you too much. It is better to have too little as it is easy to add more, but once it is in you can't take it out.

☆ Botox is also used for treating stress-related headaches. In fact, one of my female patients who had botox treatment for

her wrinkles was amazed to discover it cured the terrible
headaches that usually accompanied her periods.

☆ Don't get botox done in a nail salon or in someone's kitchen.
Always ensure a doctor is present.

☆ Women are more pain-sensitive when they have got their
period. If you are going to have injections, avoid this time.

☆ In February 2006 the UK government officially approved the
cosmetic use of botox but under the name of Vistabel.

Where on the body?

☆ Best for frown area, crow's feet and wrinkles at the top of the
nose.

☆ On the neck it is useful for the vertical bands that go from jaw
line to collarbone and the horizontal necklace lines.

☆ On the mouth it can be used to lessen deep smoker's lines or
nose-to-lip lines and downturn at the corners of the mouth,
but it is risky in these areas – there is a fine line between a
good result and side-effects. The side-effects are wonky
smiles, and weak lip muscles that can't suck on a straw or
close firmly enough to stop you dribbling. So take care here.

☆ Irregular chin.

☆ Excessive hand and underarm sweating.

☆ Headaches.

Common myths

Botox freezes all facial expressions, leaving you looking blank.

Provided you go to an experienced cosmetic doctor, you will still be able to smile, laugh and scowl at the boss but your lines will be less noticeable.

You must not fly for a week after having botox.

This myth comes from a press story about a woman who caught a plane soon after she had had botox. Shortly after landing she discovered one of her eyebrows had drooped, which she blamed on the change in air pressure. This is highly unlikely – the person who treated her had simply overdone it on the botox.

Botox stays in the body forever, damaging vital organs.

Not true. Though the effects last several months, studies show botox is eliminated from the body after two to four weeks.

The 'botox delay' – people register emotion too late.

An urban myth concocted by gossip columnists.

You can get botulism from botox injections.

No. We are giving less than one hundredth of what would give you botulism, and botox attaches to the muscle's nerve messenger within a few hours. Any excess toxin is eliminated from the body through its waste system.

Some people are resistant to botox.

I have only seen this where patients have had large doses of botox for medical reasons, for example back or neck spasms. This makes botox less effective if they want it for cosmetic reasons.

You can get creams that relax wrinkles.

There are no creams that can relax the muscles like botox. Everything we have seen so far is founded on pseudo-science. The claims don't make sense – the molecules are too big to be absorbed. The moisturizer plumps up the skin temporarily, but that is all. Apparently there is a seaweed product that supposedly relaxes muscle – what a load of Faux Tox!

Does it hurt?

It doesn't need an anaesthetic. My patients say it doesn't hurt and any discomfort is short-lived because it is quick. Some very sensitive patients could ask for a topical anaesthetic cream.

Andrea

Before a treatment I remove any makeup from the areas where the doctor does the injections and sit propped up on the couch. I have to smile and frown so the doctor can see where he needs to put the botox in, but I relax my face for the injecting part. Each injection lasts about three seconds. If I feel any discomfort at all, it is when he does the ones just under my eyes, but it is so quick it doesn't bother me.

He does a few on my temples, a couple between my eyebrows and three or four around the outside edges of my eyes. He gives me a cool-pack to hold against the bits he injected, to prevent little bruises from the needle-pricks. And the cool-pack has some paper towel wrapped around it to blot the tiny specks of blood made by the injections. The whole thing lasts about ten minutes but it flies because we are busy chatting and I'm fiddling around with the ice-pack.

Before I walk out onto the street, I wait ten minutes for any redness to go down. And I don't put my makeup back on for three to four hours because this is how long it takes for the little needle-pricks to heal over.

At first I don't feel or see any difference wrinkle-wise, but a few days later I sense a slight resistance when I scrunch up my face. A week later, although I can still smile and frown, it is more difficult to make deep furrows and lines. This lasts about four months on me, and then I feel the muscles getting stronger and see more pleats under my eyes when I smile, and I know it is time for a top-up.

I'm really pleased. The crow's feet around my eyes have completely gone, and they haven't come back because I keep going for top-ups. I look calmer and more relaxed. They say smiling makes you feel happy, and I feel the same way about not being able to furrow my brow – it makes me feel less anxious.

I've been using botox for about three years now. It is part of my general effort to look good, like wearing makeup or colouring my hair. My tip for anyone thinking about trying botox for wrinkles is that the unnatural, all-smooth look is avoidable if you go to an expert – I didn't realize that before I had it.

Eleanor

Two years ago I started sweating under my arms – really badly. I'm 48 so it's probably the menopause but it wasn't just the embarrassment – I run a high-profile business so it really hampered my work. Then I just happened to take a glance at my friend's copy of the *Daily Mail* and saw an article about botox for sweating. I read it and thought I'd give it a try.

I'm a sceptic normally, but I have to say I think botox is brilliant. I started having it last year. Once I'd chatted with the doctor and checked that it didn't go into your bloodstream, etc., I decided to go ahead. He did a test with talc and iodine to see where to put the injections. It wasn't painful – just a few pinpricks – and within 20 minutes of going in I was out again. It took about a week to work but then it lasted five months.

It's the best thing I ever did. Bad sweating is very embarrassing, especially if you have to look good for your job. My tip? Just don't worry. If you sweat profusely, get it done.

Facial

Chemical

Peels

What they are

Peels are chemical potions that are painted on the skin in order to exfoliate it. The earliest peel, used to treat acne scarring in the 1930s, was very strong and irritating, but today peels are available in much milder strengths. The strength depends on how acidic the chemical is and how long it is left on, a bit like hair highlights.

Light peels

Glycolic acid, a naturally occurring acid from sugar cane, is a good example of a gentle chemical peel. It 'unglues' the dead skin cells so they wipe off, revealing newer skin underneath that has a more even tone and texture because it has not been exposed to the elements. It is a common beauty-salon treatment and should not feel uncomfortable unless your skin is extra-sensitive.

Expect sun spots to fade and your skin to look more radiant. The light, superficial peels are much more potent than a facial scrub or loofah, but they can't reduce fixed scars or fine lines like a medium peel can. For a month after a superficial peel the skin feels nice and moist to touch, and if you have them monthly for six months your skin gets firmer, because it is producing more collagen.

Medium peels

These peels go deeper, so they improve wrinkles and reduce acne scars and blotches, but as these peels effectively use acid to burn the skin in a controlled way there is a week or two of downtime while the new skin reforms. During the first couple of weeks the skin peels off, swells, looks red and feels hot and tight, as if you have had sunburn. After this you can get out and about but you will need to cover up with makeup because your skin will still be red and shiny for three more weeks.

Examples of medium peels are:

☆ TCA (trichloroacetic acid)
☆ Jessners
☆ Low-percentage phenol

Deep peels

Strong peels are hardly used at all now – they have had their day. They literally peel off the skin down to the deeper layers to reduce scarring, age spots and wrinkles. They were used for skin resurfacing before we had lasers to do this. Lasers are better because they are easier to control – once you have painted the acid on you can't halt the process like you can with a laser.

Despite this, some practitioners do still use strong peels, but I don't and I don't recommend them. The side-effects include skin infections and cold sores, persisting redness, lasting scarring, dark patches and loss of pigment.

 Tips

☆ Before and after peels, only use products your doctor has recommended.

☆ Using Retin-A too soon after a peel can make your skin red and scaly. If it is part of your skincare routine, ask your doctor to tell you when it is safe to reintroduce it.

☆ You mustn't sun yourself for at least two weeks after a superficial peel and for up to three months after a deep peel.

How they work

The facial scrubs you can buy in the shops remove dead and flaky skin, making your complexion smoother and brighter. Peels work in the same way but they go deeper, so you see a more noticeable and longer-term improvement in your complexion. The deeper you go, the more layers of skin you remove and the bigger and quicker the improvement. However, the further down you go, the longer it takes for your skin to recover. So it is about striking a balance between getting the effect you are looking for and not irritating your skin too much. You and your doctor can decide what effect you are after and choose the right peel for the job.

 Tip

☆ Toners are a waste of time and money – they don't do anything and those that contain alcohol can dry your skin or send it into oil-producing overdrive.

How effective are they?

There is no straightforward answer to this. Medium-strength peels give a more marked improvement than light peels but involve more downtime. Don't expect overnight miracles from a superficial peel, but the benefit is they don't interrupt your routine.

Skin fitness

You exercise your muscles to keep fit. Peels, microderm-abrasion and light treatments all stimulate your skin in a similar way. By getting the skin to turn over a bit faster, you are keeping your immune system fit and the elastic fibres and collagen in your skin healthy and strong.

Where on the body?

Mainly the face and neck, but superficial peels are also popular on the hands.

 Tips

☆ The neck skin is so thin and sensitive that I have even seen superficial peels cause neck burns.

☆ If you have used a new skin product or been out in the sun the skin becomes more sensitive, so always tell the doctor what skin creams you have been using.

☆ Don't have peels if your skin has recently been exposed to the sun or if you have tanned or naturally dark skin – you are more likely to get dark or pale blotches.

☆ Peels are not suitable for people with sensitive skin, broken skin or an inflammatory skin condition like eczema or dermatitis. There are a host of skin conditions that rule out peels for you and the doctor should check for these before treating you.

☆ Red light or IPL are good alternatives to peels if you have sensitive skin.

Holly

I've had two courses of light glycolic peels. At the moment I'm on my third course of six. I decided to try them to improve the texture of my skin, which is bumpy and uneven from damage and spots when I was younger.

When I go in, I lie on the couch and the therapist puts a towel over my hair. Before she puts the peel on, she cleanses my face and tones it with some alcohol solution. Then she smears on the peel mixture in circular movements with a giant cotton bud.

It feels a bit itchy and tingly but the therapist makes it more comfortable by gently and constantly massaging my face. The first time I had it done they only left the peel on for five minutes, but each time I go they leave it on a bit longer. To take it off they use bicarbonate of soda because it neutralizes the acid. Then they moisturize my face and I can put my makeup on straight away. Once I went out for the day straight after I'd had a peel, but I usually prefer to book an evening session so I can go home afterwards to relax.

One evening before I went to have a peel, I rushed home from work, jumped in the shower and, without thinking, gave my face a really thorough scrub with those little grains you can buy. Two minutes after the lady started putting the peel on my face started stinging, so I told her and she took the peel off straight away – she was very quick. The peel felt sore because I'd made my skin quite raw with the scrub. For a couple of days afterwards my face was a bit swollen and I had little scabs, like carpet burns, on my temples, under my eyes and underneath my chin. It went down after a couple of days but it gave me a bit of a shock, so I'd advise people not to put other products on their face before having a peel, or if they do they should let the therapist know.

Occasionally I get a little bit of dryness and some tiny, tiny pinhead blisters around my mouth, but as you have more treatments you get to know your sensitive areas and you and the therapist can adjust the treatment to allow for them.

The recommended number of sessions is a course of six, but I found I needed more. Before I had my first one, they took a photo under one of those nasty lights that shows up all the damage – it looked horrible – then after I'd had six sessions they did this again. I could see slight improvements on certain areas but I decided to book more sessions to get it looking better.

My skin feels so much smoother now that I'm going to stop at the end of this course and just have maintenance sessions. My advice to anyone going to have a peel is to just relax. The worst part is not knowing what to expect.

Endermology

How it works

This is a non-invasive method of treating diffused, localized or flabby cellulite.

It was originally devised for injuries to muscles, but it is now used in clinics and beauty salons as a high-tech way of massaging the skin to improve the appearance of cellulite. It has a hand-piece with two rollers on it that you roll up and down on the skin, while a sucker in between the rollers draws the skin up. It kneads the skin much more vigorously than a therapist could with his or her bare hands.

After liposuction, patients can be left with lumps, and this treatment is sometimes performed to reduce these. However, it is mainly used to treat cellulite and works best on surface cellulite in younger people. It will not make a big difference to established cellulite in more mature women where the cellulite is fixed, i.e. lumpy and visible when all muscles are relaxed. So have realistic expectations.

You need to be dedicated to get results: initial treatment involves twice-weekly sessions for six weeks and then maintenance sessions every three months. It takes a session of around 45 minutes to massage the whole body, and you will need to eat the right things and take regular exercise – it is not going to work on its own.

Side-effects

The worst thing that could happen is a bruise, but this can only happen if the machine is set too high. If it feels uncomfortable, let the therapist know.

Where on the body?

All over the body, but more work will be done on the buttocks and thighs, where cellulite appears.

Common myths

Powerful electronic massages can make you lose weight.
False: Endermology is not a slimming machine.

Does it hurt?

You wear a body stocking, so the sucking action doesn't pinch the skin. The treatment pressure is quite intense but it shouldn't be uncomfortably painful. If it is hurting, you have it set too high and this could give you bruises. Ask for the power to be turned down.

Emma

I came across endermology ten years ago in France, which is where I've spent most of my adult life, and I've been using it ever since. In my mid-twenties I noticed I was bloating out, but I couldn't understand why. I ate well and did loads of exercise – I used to run every day – but in the end I discovered it was because I had bad circulation, which runs in my family. It was giving me bloating and horrible cellulite.

Endermology is a popular treatment in France, and a lot of physiotherapists offer it. I found it really worked for me, especially on my legs. I had it really intensively and it changed everything. My skin got clearer and I felt a lot better. I also ate well and walked a lot – I'm quite strong-willed. It's got to be combined with keeping active. When I was active it would last for a month. People would look at me and could see the difference.

This last year I've been living in the UK, working in an office where I'm sitting down for the most of the day, and with one thing and another I've also had less endermology treatments. I've noticed a lot of the bloating has come back. I'm slim and I have a small frame but I still have localized cellulite. I know a lot of people have endermology done for aesthetic reasons, and I do too, but it's not just the appearance that bothers me – I hate the way my legs feel heavy and tired. I find it harder to be healthy in the UK, with all this rubbish food available and the awful weather.

When I have the treatment it feels like a really intense massage. It's very powerful – much more powerful than a hand massage – and it massages a much bigger area. It's like a roller with a really heavy suction action and it lifts up the layers of skin. It feels like it is breathing life into the cells. It's very good for cellulite – you can feel a slight increase in pressure when it goes over the lumps, but it doesn't hurt. There are different strengths so you can always stop the therapist and have it changed.

When it has finished you can feel the blood circulating. You can tell it's done you good. You walk out feeling lighter. It's invigorating. But you will want to go to the loo straight away!

☆ *Emma's tips*

☆ Have it three times a week at the beginning to trigger the system.

☆ It is not a quick fix, it is a long-term treatment, but it is worth it.

☆ Don't be embarrassed about getting undressed and wearing a body stocking.

☆ It makes you want to go to the toilet, so visit the loo beforehand.

☆ Get photos done and then compare three months later, so you can see how your skin has got smoother.

☆ Be prepared to eat healthily and drink lots of water to flush out the toxins, particularly at the beginning of the treatment.

Fillers

How they work

Fillers act like padding you can place under the skin in small amounts, using a needle. Until the end of the 1990s, collagen was the only filler available, apart from silicone, but silicone has serious side-effects.

Collagen injections (derived from cattle skin) have been around since the 1970s, and they are still one of only a small selection of fillers available in the US because they have a different system for regulating medical products that requires long-term testing. Collagen is not long-lasting but it can give you an allergic reaction.

However, in the early 1990s non-animal-sourced fillers came along. There are loads of these and new ones are being introduced all the time, so it is very confusing. There are about 70 available in the European Union, but I would recommend the temporary hyaluronic-acid fillers.

Six to twelve months temporary fillers

Hyaluronic acid, which occurs naturally in skin and cartilage, has been used in fillers for ten years. These fillers have been fully researched, so we know they are safe and don't contain ingredients that give you allergic reactions. They can last up to a year or more, but it varies from person to person and from one area of the face to another. At the moment, the best fillers are the temporary ones, because although it would be good if a filler lasted two to three years, those that currently do can give you long-lasting problems including an allergic reaction.

The only side-effect of hyaluronic, which occurs once in every 5,000 patients, is a low-grade allergy that amounts to a bit of redness for three to four weeks, which can be covered up with makeup. So it is nothing serious. Most patients get a bit of swelling because hyaluronic acid attracts water to itself, but this is slight and only lasts for a few days.

One to two year long-term fillers

Longer-term versions are made of little granules mixed in with the hyaluronic acid or collagen. These silicone-type granules are designed to stay in the body longer, but they can cause an allergic reaction, which is what happened to Leslie Ash. If you try a long-term filler and this happens to you, you have to have steroid injections and it will take years to go. I have had people turn up with this problem in various areas of their face. It looks lumpy and red. It comes and goes but the filler is designed to stay there, so the problem lasts a long time. Therefore, if a filler is claiming to last for one to two years, my advice is to be cautious.

Permanent fillers

Silicone or gortex are permanent fillers, but they can produce permanent problems. I've seen people with lumps, particularly in the lips, and some cases where the silicone has moved to another area. There are no real options to reduce lumps other than surgery to actually cut it out, and even if you don't have any of these problems and it looks great, when you are older and the skin around it droops it is going to look unnatural.

Grow your own

As an alternative to fillers, some practitioners are offering patients the option of cultivating their own collagen-producing cells and having them reinserted wherever their skin needs plumping to reduce wrinkles. A bit of skin is taken from behind their ear and sent off to a lab, where it is used to grow the cells. Once enough have grown, the cells are returned and implanted.

The idea sounds fantastic and it may work somehow in the future, but at the moment it is not foolproof and it is extremely expensive. Often the collagen-producing cells fail to grow in the lab. Then those that do grow fail to grow any collagen once they are implanted. Occasionally and surprisingly, an allergy may occur: something they do in the lab changes the cells, giving the patient an adverse reaction that can last for up to three months. So I would say this method still needs a bit of fine-tuning, exciting though it is.

Where on the body?

☆ lips and smoker's lines
☆ nose-to-lip lines
☆ secondary smile lines on the cheek
☆ corners of the mouth where they droop down
☆ frown lines and forehead
☆ crow's feet
☆ depressed scars
☆ hollow cheeks
☆ lost volume in cheeks

Do they hurt?

All fillers are injected, so there will be a degree of discomfort, but you can have a topical anaesthetic or a dental block. If you are being injected round your cheeks or eyes then the cream is enough, but lip injections are more uncomfortable, so a dental block is best.

There is a little channel where the skin meets the lip, and injecting filler into this channel produces a tidy rim. When injecting into the pink of the lip it can go lumpy because it can move around and collect into areas, especially when you are talking – so gently massage the area where you have had filler put in to keep things smooth. Do this three times a day for about seven days. After a week it is unlikely that massage will make any difference because the filler integrates with the skin. Gradually the immune system and mechanical movement break it down, and because it is a naturally occurring thing it just gets absorbed and you go back to how you were.

Pat

Five years ago I started to get depressed when I looked in the mirror. I thought, I don't look good any more. It was an overnight thing. I tried creams but they didn't really work. I thought, skin creams aren't going to do enough – and they're not cheap. I'd read about things you could have done in magazines but didn't know where to go, and then I told my friend I was thinking about having something done and she said, 'I go to a guy. Why don't you try him?' I never knew my friend had had anything done; she'd never let on.

I was quite nervous, so I took my friend for backup and advice. I lay on a dentist's couch and looked into a big mirror while he suggested what he could do. I got excited. I thought, this is just what I want, and I relaxed because I felt confident in him.

I had Restylane around my mouth, jowl lines, and under and on top of my lips. When he did the injections it hurt. Nearest my nose was the worst bit, but I put up with it. It's not nice to have injections in your face, but it doesn't make you cry or anything and it's just for a few seconds, that's all. The lips were fine because he numbed those. I don't think anyone could stand injections in their lips otherwise.

I was amazed. It made me feel good. He took a photo before he did it and six months later he showed it to me, and that was when I realized what a difference it had made. The effects have lasted so long. I've only had it done twice. When I had my lips done the second time I got my husband to pick me up because my lips get very swollen, but after two days they looked fabulous. Now the top lip matches the bottom!

People say, 'Oh, you look great today,' but I don't tell anyone. I say I've had my hair done. As far as I know I'm the only girl at work who has contemplated it. I don't tell my kids but my husband knows. He's happy that I'm happy and he likes me looking good. I think Restylane is a wonderful treatment because it's a natural product and it's safe. I like not looking my age. I know it is a bit shallow and people say you should grow old gracefully, but I think that's a load of [beep!]. If it makes you happy, why not?

Intense Pulsed Light (IPL)

What it is

One IPL system is pretty much the same as another. They are versatile machines. They remove hair, particularly well on those with fairer skin types and darker hairs; they can remove broken veins from the face; they can be used to calm the redness of acne rosacea; they can fade sun spots and pigmentation brought about by sun damage; and they can be used to rejuvenate skin, making it firmer by stimulating the growth of new collagen. They have a slight edge over lasers when it comes to hair removal because they can cover a larger area more quickly.

They are not so good at reducing wrinkles, birthmarks or tattoos (for the latter they don't work at all).

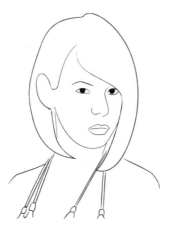

How it works

IPL works in a similar way to lasers, but because it can
search for more colours it can find and remove brown and
red hair. And you can adjust the setting so the same machine
that removes hair can be used for skin rejuvenation.

You see a bright, momentary flash from the hand-piece as
it is held against the area being treated. This is the very
intense light that is being directed down a tube to find the
pigment you want it to work on. It is very quick. Then you
move the hand-piece to the next area you want to treat and
give that a burst of light, and so on.

 Tip

☆ Expect it to be briefly uncomfortable when the machine
goes 'flash'. The cooling device on the system is a blast of
cold air that is used to cool your skin down first, so the flash
feels less hot. Some just use an ice-pack, but a cooling device
will make you more comfortable.

Side-effects

There is a slim risk of burning if the skin is tanned, dark or flushed. The light gets confused and heats the colour in your skin instead of the hair or spider vein you want it to heat. But you can avoid this if you have the treatment when you don't have a suntan or a flushed face, and the practitioner can adjust the settings down to allow for extra colour in your skin. (This may mean you require more sessions, but it is better than giving you a burn.)

 Tips

☆ Make sure you remove all your makeup before a session of IPL, or the light will target the makeup colour and frazzle it.

☆ I see advertisements for IPL tattoo removal, but I'm afraid this does not work.

☆ If you have grey or blonde hairs, IPL will not remove them.

Where on the body?

Hair and skin all over, but predominantly the treatments are on the sun-exposed areas: the face, neck, hands, chest and shoulders. The most common areas for hair removal are the underarm and bikini line.

Caroline

I went into the clinic to ask about cosmeceutical creams, but when I was having my consultation the doctor said, 'You've got a bit of rosacea there.' I didn't know what rosacea was, but when he described the symptoms – a red nose, little red spots, broken blood vessels, sensitive flushed skin that gets worse when you have a coffee – I thought, yes, this is me, but I hadn't realized these things were symptoms of a skin condition. I just thought I had a naturally rubbish complexion. I was pleased to hear there was something I could do to change it.

When I had to lie down on the couch, surrounded by all this equipment, I felt nervous, but once the doctor started chatting to me I calmed down. The nurse used a spatula to put cold gel on my face and gave me a pair of tinted goggles. She held a tube that was blowing out chilled air close to my cheek. Then, through my goggles I saw a bright flash that made me jump. I felt a sharp but short whipping pain, which hurt, but only briefly. It hurt more on my cheeks than on my nose and chin.

The doctor worked his way across the affected areas of my face, allowing the nurse to cool the area first each time, before he flashed the light. The whole thing took about ten minutes, after which I cleaned off the gel, put some makeup on and went off to pick the kids up from school. My face felt a bit warm for a few hours but then I'm used to that.

After two weeks my skin had really calmed down and my broken veins were disappearing, and by the end of the third week I felt really excited about how much better it looked. I couldn't wait to go back for my next session, and that made it improve even more.

Now my face feels much more comfortable, I don't have embarrassing flushes all the time and it takes me half as long to get ready in the morning because I don't have to camouflage myself in an inch of makeup. My cheeks look really good – not just a more even colour but smoother and firmer too. Several friends have commented on it.

I'm a real fan. My husband says I look better now, in my thirties, than I did in my twenties. I think a lot of people probably have rosacea and don't realize. If you think you do, get it checked out, then try the IPL: the difference is amazing. And when you have the treatment, ask if you can hold the cooler yourself. Use it to make your skin as cold as you comfortably can, then tell your practitioner when you are ready for him to zap – and don't point it up your nose because that takes your breath away!

Lasers

What they are

Lasers are useful for all kinds of things in medicine and surgery. The first lasers for skin problems were developed in the 1960s, to remove birthmarks – both brown ones and the red ones that are commonly called port-wine stains. Now there are loads of different types of lasers, all specifically designed to deal with particular cosmetic problems.

How they work

Lasers are colour biased. They send out a single wavelength of light that is only interested in one colour. It ignores the other colours and passes through them. When it finds the one it is looking for it goes into it and heats it up.

In the way a microwave heats up the food but not the container, you could use a laser to heat a tomato through a piece of cling film. The tomato would disintegrate but the cling film would be left untouched. It is quite high-tech.

No-surgery trivia question to test your friends:

Q. What does LASER stand for?

A. Light Amplification by Stimulated Emission of Radiation

What they do

Lasers that remove wrinkles

These lasers are used for skin resurfacing. They burn the skin off in a controlled way. This type smoothes out wrinkles, lines and creases, micro-layer by micro-layer.

Lasers that plump the skin

These work by heating up the collagen to stir it into growing new collagen (there are lots of these and they are all the same).

Lasers to remove broken blood vessels

The heat from the laser seals the blood vessel off from the rest of the blood vessels, so the body recognizes it as something it doesn't need any more and carries it off to be disposed as waste. Lasers are good for removing small vessels, but if it is thread veins on legs you want to get rid of, microsclerotherapy works better.

Lasers that remove hair

The heat from these lasers seeks out brown and black (so they don't see blonde and grey hair). When it finds the brown or black hair, the heat goes down the hair shaft into the follicle to destroy it. As hairs grow in cycles every four to six weeks, you will not get them all first time. You have to laser each cycle of hair growth. You usually get about a third of them at any one time, so you will need a minimum of three or four sessions to get the best result. There are lasers that are designed specifically for darker skins.

Lasers that remove tattoos

These work by transferring heat into the colour to explode the pigment and disperse it. The immune system finds the leftover pigment debris, tidies it up and carries it away to dispose of it.

Pigment lasers

These remove sun spots using a similar method to tattoo lasers.

Lasers for birthmarks

These are more powerful lasers that go deep into the skin. They go into the pigment of the birthmark and seal the blood vessels, which makes the birthmark fade. But these are large blood vessels so it takes more than ten sessions, feels quite sore, and takes up to six weeks to heal.

Mary on smoker's lines and laser resurfacing

I had these very pronounced lines above my lips because I used to be a heavy smoker, years ago. I'm not a nervous person and when I heard I could get them done I thought, why not. They really didn't look very nice and they were very deep.

It felt a bit uncomfortable – like a hot needle. The doctor said, 'How does that feel? Can you bear it if I turn it up a bit higher to make it more effective?' I thought, well, this is nothing much really, better than having all those lines, so I said he could. I came out of the clinic and went to M&S to meet my daughter. I had this gel on my face but I was feeling fine.

It takes the skin off, so it was sore for a night, like I'd burned myself badly in the sun. Then that wore off and it just looked red for a little while. I can imagine it would be more painful if they did it on your whole face, but because I just had a small bit done I could cover it up quite easily with a bit of powder.

To a friend I would say 'be calm'. People go through the most horrendous things to look good, but this wasn't too painful at all. I went back to work the next day, but I wouldn't have gone out in the evening.

This was five years ago and it is still much better than it was, so it was really worth having it done. I'm 70, and people still say I don't look my age. I've thought about a facelift but I'm a bit squeamish about that, and then I'd have to start on the rest of my body, wouldn't I?

Anne on laser resurfacing

I'm 58 now. Because I lived in Africa for many years I got a lot of lines. I saw this laser-resurfacing treatment advertised, and it was mainly the pigmentation I wanted to get rid of. I wanted to even the tone of my skin and lose some of the lines. I needed my whole face done.

Once the doctor talked me through what would happen, I went and sat on a dentist's chair and put these goggles on for most of it – he removed them for my eyes. The nurse had a little tube to clean up any residue. It felt hot. First it was like an elastic band across your face, but as it got deeper, it hurt more. I've got a high pain threshold so it must have been quite bad. Even with anaesthetic it still hurt. I thought, I can put up with this, and then I started to find it quite painful. Towards the end I thought, I can't go on. It lasted about an hour and a half but it felt like a long time.

Afterwards my face looked as if someone had thrown a bucket of boiling water over it. Then I had to clean it with a solution of water with vinegar before covering it with a mixture of Vaseline and white paraffin, to keep out the air and germs. The doctor told me this made it heal without scabbing so the new skin grows smoothly. I looked like the Bride of Dracula for a little while. People would have looked at me in shock and horror if I'd gone out. I had to bathe it every four hours and then put Vaseline on. It was weepy and the discomfort kept me awake the first couple of nights. The first few days I thought, what did I do this for? Is it going to look any better?

But after about a week the redness calmed down and I could see there were less lines and there was less pigmentation. Because I could see it was working, I started to feel more upbeat. Then when it healed it looked smoother and better all over. It was a really good psychological boost.

This was about five years ago now, and it's wearing off a little bit. To a friend I would say go for it, because to me it's a better option than surgery, but in this day and age there might be alternatives. I am really pleased with the results, but talking about it now, I'm glad it's behind me.

Light Treatments

How they work

These are relatively recent additions to the range of no-surgery treatments.

The light you get from a light bulb is made up of lots of different colours of lights combined. You can see all these different colours in a rainbow. The red and blue lights are used in skin rejuvenation because they can penetrate the skin without damaging its surface and without any discomfort, to do good work on its under-layers. Red is a skin rejuvenator. It makes your skin look healthy, firmer, plumper and glowing. Infrared light speeds up healing, and blue light kills bacteria in the skin, so it is used to treat spots. These are very popular treatments. Patients who try them always return for more.

My ideal beauty treatment... one that makes me look great instantly, yet doesn't take all afternoon.

Julia Carling on red light

Red light

Red light is used as a no-surgery skin rejuvenation treatment.
It gives the skin an instant radiance that lasts for three to five
days, and if you have several treatments it plumps up the skin
long-term. It improves the condition of the skin, increasing
cell activity. This is a great treatment to have just before a
special event or to encourage the skin to heal quickly.

 Tip

☆ The light may seem very bright, but it doesn't harm your
eyes, so lie back and relax! The light will make you feel better,
particularly in the depths of winter.

Near infrared light

Near infrared is the red light that is used in your telly
controls. It doesn't feel hot like far infrared and you can't
see or feel it. It penetrates the skin slightly further than red
light, where it stimulates the kind of collagen that stays
around in your skin long-term. So this is good for scarring
and wrinkles. It has been used for a few years to speed up
the healing process after surgery, and now it has become
available as a no-surgery treatment for scarring and wrinkles.
You need a course of treatments to get the full effect.

☆ *Tip*

☆ As for red light, enjoy it – it is relaxing, and it is doing you good.

Cost: Expect to pay £60 per session.

Patient pain rating: 1 (1– 10, 1=pain-free)

Treatment Time: Needs 3 treatments per week for 3 weeks running to get the skin in optimum condition.

How long does it last? Up to 3 months, but just have maintenance sessions when you feel you need them.

Blue light

This is good for spots and oily skin. Blue light penetrates two to three millimetres into the skin, targeting the layers at hair-follicle level, where it kills harmful bacteria. It takes a series of treatments to work. Initially, the skin gets worse, but by week four patients usually start to see and feel the improvement. Expect to see between 70–80 per cent improvement.

This is a good alternative to taking antibiotics. Apart from making the skin a little bit pink for an hour, it doesn't have any side-effects. Some drugs, medical conditions and the herbal remedy St John's wort can make you light sensitive, but your practitioner will always check these things out before he treats you.

Cost: £350 for a course of 8 sessions, 2 per week, for 4 weeks.

Patient pain rating: 1 (1– 10, 1=pain-free)

Treatment time: 30 minutes

How long does it last? This is a maintenance programme. It varies from person to person, but the benefits can last up to 6 months.

 Tips

☆ You need to allow 48 hours between different coloured-light treatments.

☆ This is a treatment you can have in a beauty salon.

☆ Red light is a good treatment to combine with no-surgery treatments that require a bit of healing time: lasers, peels or microdermabrasion.

☆ Red light is a good treatment to get the skin's healing and immune systems firing on all cylinders before surgery.

Where on the body?

Light treatments can be used on any part of the body. Red light is used for rejuvenation anywhere, but usually on the face. Infrared is used to promote scar healing anywhere on the body. Blue light is used on the back or chest, but mostly on the face.

Alison

I'm a police officer. I never had acne when I was a kid, it started in my late thirties, and it was dreadful. I had a face like a pizza and I couldn't do anything about it. Makeup just highlighted it. When I was at work I think people must have looked and thought, Don't mention it, she'll pan me.

I tried topical solutions and zinc scrubs, and everything the NHS can offer, including Roaccutane – twice – but it gave me very dry skin and dry lips. I wasn't allowed in the sun, I was repeatedly told not to get pregnant and I found it quite scary. I don't think it did anything for me. All in all I had ten years of treatment but nothing worked. I just thought, Why, why? It made me terribly self-conscious. Rather than wanting to look younger, I just wanted to look normal. Some people said things like 'You'll grow out of it' or 'Too many chips', but the worst moment was when I visited my doctor, who wasn't very understanding and said, 'At least it's only on your face.' Only on your face!? Now, I am not a blubber, but at that point, I have to admit, I broke down.

I looked into alternatives and I was planning to try a few no-surgery treatments, like lasers and things, but the first one I tried was blue light, which I had alongside antibiotics. I had eight treatments. They felt comfortable, quite relaxing actually. I just had to put some goggles on and wait for about fifteen minutes and that is all I remember. I had a little redness afterwards, but no pain. When it's improved, you forget how bad you looked, until you see the pictures. Looking at the pictures I can really see the difference. I still have scarring and need to wear makeup, but it is much better; I would say I had a 75 per cent improvement.

To someone else I would say it was a time in my life when I was stressed. I was going through a divorce and I was working hard on a course. It felt like everything was going wrong and these factors may have been partly responsible for the acne getting so bad. This is going to sound like one of those true-life stories, but since my skin has improved I've lost three and a half stone and got a new fella.

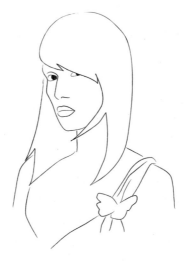

Pia and Don

Pia: My husband and I love this treatment regularly. I have to take my jewellery off and we lie on beds with our heads on cushions. Our faces are cleaned, we put some goggles on and they put a band around my hair. Then the very strong bright light is switched on, very close to your face. We keep our eyes closed. It feels very warm, not hot, and we lie there for about 20 minutes while the beautician massages our arms and hands and we chat quietly.

Afterwards we have moisturizer put on and look in the mirror. You can see you are glowing and your skin looks soft. I can see a difference in the softening of the lines around my eyes, which don't look as deep. It's a very nice feeling. Our skin looks plump and glowing for four or five days, and our friends say, 'You look so healthy.' I can see it in my husband – everything is softer and he looks healthy, as if he's been in the sun or on a long walk. The glowing doesn't last more than a couple of days, but we do see a longer-lasting improvement. When we first came for the treatment we had photos taken, and when we compare them to some photos we had taken after we'd been having the treatment for a few months, the lines are not as deep.

Don: When I sit in the waiting room I feel a bit self-conscious, but once I'm in the treatment clinic I feel fine, and the light feels pleasantly warm and the time seems to go pretty quickly. You've got goggles but the machine is quite close to your face, so I prefer to keep my eyes closed. I think most people would.

They take Polaroids so you can see the difference. I always joke about the photos because Polaroids make such terrible pictures – you couldn't look worse if you tried – but I can see the improvements. When we come back home we laugh because we're both over 60 and we've got this lovely glowing pink skin.

It's an ego thing, I suppose – a confidence booster. We look after ourselves, and we go to a gym, and people say we don't look our ages, which makes you feel good. When people look at me they see a pensioner. I'm 77, but they don't realize that I'm not 77 inside – I still think and feel as I did when I was 30. When people say you look well, it cheers you up. The plumping doesn't last but we go back every few weeks because it makes us feel good again, and it isn't dangerous or bad for the skin, like a sun lamp. I would recommend it.

Minor Surgery

What it is

Things that can be sliced or shaved with a local anaesthetic make for a relatively easy procedure because they don't need stitching, but we can cut out and stitch up unwanted lumps and bumps in the space of a lunchtime, provided they are not too large. When it is a mole, however, because there are so many different types I can't give you general guidelines. Before you get a mole removed for cosmetic reasons, you need to get it checked by a GP or dermatologist, to make sure it is benign.

Who does it?

If it is purely cosmetic you can see a private doctor who is trained in these procedures: a private GP, a surgeon or a cosmetic doctor. If it is on your face, however, the choice narrows down to either a plastic surgeon or an experienced cosmetic doctor, because a GP will be wary of removing lumps and bumps on the face.

☆ *Tips*
  ☆ Only allow the freezing treatments if there is no alternative, because they leave pale white marks.

☆ Eat a varied diet and use creams containing vitamin E and C to help the skin heal nicely.

Side-effects

There will always be a little mark that fades over time. And in a few cases the scar can stretch and get bigger, or get infected, or go lumpy. These things are rare, but you should talk to your practitioner about the chances of anything like this.

What to expect

What we are looking to do is keep the scarring and marking to a minimum. If you have a flat mark instead of a raised lump it is easier to conceal.

Sheila

I had this mole for a long time above my right eyebrow. It started to bother me when my other half mentioned it and when I saw it in photos. I knew it wasn't cancerous but I decided to get it seen to – it was just vanity really. I asked the cosmetic doctor whether he could remove it, and after taking a look he said this wouldn't be a problem at all.

He injected me with a local anaesthetic and after that I couldn't really tell what was going on. I just heard him say, 'You're a vascular little thing, aren't you.' I needed five stitches and I have to admit that when I first saw it in the mirror it looked a bit ugly. Then it went a bit weepy for a few days, but after that I was really surprised at how it suddenly improved. It's healed amazingly now and I'm really pleased it's gone.

I think it's important to be absolutely sure you want it done. My advice to others is don't panic when you first see it: be prepared for the fact it will look a mess immediately afterwards, but give it a week and it will look much better.

Lotions and Potions

It's confusing, isn't it? We seem to get daily announcements from cosmetic companies about new miracle creams that can smooth away wrinkles, cellulite, spots, etc. Do they work? And if they do, how do you recall which one it was you wanted to try? There are so many and they all have similar-sounding, science-speak names you can't remember. And when you get to the counter the assistant will suggest a few more.

You can't go by what it says on the packet. If you can manage to read it without a magnifying glass, you will see reams of scientific jargon that only a chemist would understand. It is a waste of your time.

So I am going to tell you about my favourite key ingredients, the ones that have undergone proper testing, the ones that have stood the test of time and that make a difference to my patients. You can get hold of them in cosmetic clinics and salons and they are referred to generally as cosmeceuticals, to distinguish them from other potions. You can't get them in the shops because they have a high concentration of ingredients. How strong the lotion or potion is affects where it is allowed to be sold. Salespeople in shops are not qualified to sell higher-strength creams because you need some dermatological (skin) know-how to make the correct skin assessment, recommend the right product and give advice on how to use it.

Pharmacists might sell some of them, but most pharmacists concentrate on stocking drugs and cosmeceuticals are not classified as drugs. These stronger cosmeceutical creams are available from clinics and salons where there are qualified therapists or doctors to ensure you have the correct product and don't give yourself a skin reaction.

Some of the ingredients are the same as those in the products you can buy in the high street, but in high-street versions you get weaker concentrations, so they are less likely to make a difference. The stronger concentrations have more of an effect but more risk of a side-effect, which is why you need someone with a bit more knowledge to tell you how to use them.

And it is not just a case of bunging together some ingredients. How they are mixed is just as important. The right ingredients need to be specially formulated to make them go to work on the skin, otherwise they would just sit there or disintegrate.

What to expect

None are going to be dramatic de-wrinklers, but they can plump up superficial layers of skin to reduce fine lines. With a cream, treatment is an ongoing process because skin turns over every month. The common theme is healthy and radiant. Don't expect miracles, but do expect them to work – we have good studies that show they do.

The top six ingredients

Glycolic acid: an excellent exfoliator and skin-smoother
Vitamin A: the skin vitamin that rejuvenates
Vitamin C: antioxidant and skin lightener
Vitamin E: antioxidant – works well with other vitamins
Coenzyme Q10: antioxidant and moisturiser
Idebenone: very powerful antioxidant – improves wrinkles

Glycolic acid

What is it? It is a fruit acid; it comes from sugar cane. There are several fruit acids used in creams, and they are collectively known as AHAs or alpha hydroxy acids. I've picked glycolic as my favourite fruit acid because I think it works the best.

What does it do? Cells replace themselves every 28 days when we are young, but this process slows up as we age to as many as 50 days. Glycolic acid gets it going again, back up to 28 days. Another thing it can do is to thin abnormally thickened skin, which is good for acne and sun damage, as well as stimulate collagen (this takes roughly six months of use), and there is scientific data to back this up! Glycolic also makes the skin absorb other products or treatments better than it would without it, so it is like a good 'mixer' in a face-cream cocktail.

What difference will it make? Plumping in six months, but most people notice their skin is softer and smoother after 1–2 weeks.

Good for: Acne, milia, sun damage, pigmentation, skin plumping.

Expect to pay: £15–£50 for a pot of cream.

Side effects: It is normal to get some tingling and a bit of redness, but if you put too much on it might give you a burning feeling, peeling and redness. So follow instructions carefully. In rare cases, some people are very sensitive to glycolic acid, so do a patch test first.

Vitamin A

What is it? In the first instance, a derivative of vitamin A known as Retin-A was introduced in the 1960s to treat acne, until one doctor noticed that several patients using Retin-A remarked on a reduction in their wrinkles. Now it is the only drug that can be prescribed for acne and/or wrinkles. The only problem with Retin-A is that it often irritates the skin, but there are other less irritating versions of vitamin A. The least irritating one I know is retinyl palmitate. Although it is not quite as strong, it is less likely to give you a reaction. Retinyl palmitate mixed with glycolic acid makes a great face-cream cocktail because they help each other work more efficiently.

What does it do? It delivers vitamin A to the cells that need it for doing skin repairs, so they work more efficiently and get more repairs done. It is good for acne, wrinkles and sun damage.

What difference will it make? After a month you should see an improvement in the texture and condition of your skin. After a good three to six months the repair mechanism should kick in. It depends on the level of damage your skin has had, but you should notice age spots fade, scars heal quicker and that your skin has more glow.

Good for: Undoing skin damage. It fades sun spots, reduces wrinkles and skin that has lost its glow because of smoking.

Expect to pay: £40+

Side-effects: Tingling and a little bit of redness is normal and shows it is working. If you use this or any vitamin A cream and go out in the sun, you are more likely to burn. But you should use a sunscreen anyway: there is no point in using a cream with vitamin A and no sunscreen if you are interested in looking after your skin – any good the cream is doing will be undone straight away by the sun.

Vitamin C

What is it? It is a powerful antioxidant, which means it intercepts skin-cell damage. It is impregnated into plasters because it speeds up wound healing. It is also used to soothe burns. Vitamin C is easily destroyed by sunlight and oxygen, so to lengthen its shelf-life it has to be mixed with things that stabilize it (on the packaging vitamin C will be listed as a derivative of ascorbic acid – for example: methyl ascorbyl phosphate).

What does it do? It does lots of things: stimulates collagen production, brightens skin (it has a slight bleaching effect), and it is anti-inflammatory.

What difference will it make? After a month of use you should notice brightening and radiance, but we are talking three to six months before you see the firming and plumping effects of increased collagen production.

Good for: Acne-scar healing, increased pigmentation and skin rejuvenation.

Expect to pay: £30+

Side-effects: Tingling and a little bit of redness are normal and show it is working.

Nugget

One ciggy destroys two oranges' worth of vitamin C.

Nugget

Zsa Zsa Gabor used to squeeze a lemon on her elbows and knees before she went to bed at night because she was mixed race and you can get dark patches (probably a build-up of dead skin). She must have got through a lot of lemons!

☆ Tip

☆ You have got to persevere with a cream. People believe you can use a product to improve the skin and then come off it, but you have got to keep at it. It is like going to the gym. Most people don't give it enough time. You need to be loyal to the routine you are advised to follow. One lady came to my clinic for cystic acne. She followed everything my therapist said and quit the sun beds. She had ten glycolic acid peels, vitamin A for repair and vitamin C to stimulate more collagen, all while her husband worked away in the forces. When he came back, she looked so different he thought she'd had a facelift.

Vitamin E

What is it? It is a protective antioxidant. It settles on the outside of our skin like bubble wrap. It is the bouncer that says, 'If your name is not down you can't come in.' It protects you from the onslaught of free radicals. These are nasty little molecules which are formed in our cells when we smoke or the sun hits the skin. They tear around the cells like bulls in a china shop causing all sorts of damage. Vitamin E helps to mop up the free radicals so the skin can repair itself in peace. It also helps to reflect UV.

What does it do? It is a protection plan – your insurance policy against skin-cell damage.

Good for: Combining with other ingredients, like vitamin C, because the two ingredients are more than twice as effective when they are working together. You could almost say: When does $1 + 1 = 2.5$? Answer: when it is 1 vitamin E + 1 vitamin C.

Expect to pay: £40. There are no useful creams that only contain vitamin E, so in a cosmeceutical cream it will always be combined with other ingredients.

Side-effects: None.

Coenzyme Q10

What is it? An antioxidant that can also speed up cell repair but using a different tactic from Retin-A.

What does it do? It provides mechanisms for the body to heal itself – what a helpful and friendly ingredient it is.

What difference does it make? After a month your skin will be functioning better so it will look healthier.

Good for: Skin rejuvenation.

Expect to pay: £40+

Side-effects: It is generally well tolerated, unless you have very sensitive skin.

Idebenone

What is it? It is used in organ transplants: if a liver was left on a theatre table it would oxidate and turn black, but if you stick it in this stuff it keeps it alive. It is given to Alzheimer patients and to children with premature-ageing syndromes.

What does it do? It stimulates collagen production. The US chemist who discovered it for beauty products is Joe Lewis, and there are independent studies that show an average of 27 per cent wrinkle-depth reduction in eight to twelve weeks. Most people notice that their skin looks better.

What difference does it make? Wrinkle reduction after eight weeks, and within three months the skin looks in better condition generally.

Good for: Fine lines and some deeper lines.

Expect to pay: £70 upwards for a product.

Side effects: A little bit of dryness and tingling.

☆ *Tip*

☆ Your skin may take a little time to adjust to the cream – this mainly applies to Retin-A but can be a problem with any strong cream. Perhaps soften the dry bits of skin with a bit of moisturizer in the meantime. It will calm down as your skin gets used to it. If you have sensitive skin then cut down and resort to on and off usage (one day on, one day off). It may take longer to get an effect, but this enables results without adverse reactions.

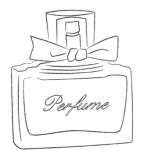

Sunscreens

Even using a sunscreen improves the skin. It allows the skin
to divert its resources to repair and renewal rather than
defending itself against sun rays. There are two types of
sunscreen: one that works by deflecting the sunlight and
another that works by absorbing it with chemicals. The
deflecting ones use either titanium dioxide or zinc oxide,
which is the silvery-white stuff in the sun blocks that skiers
paint across their noses, but the latest sunscreens use very
fine particles so you get the benefit of the protection
without the war-paint look. The absorbing ones use
oxybenzone and octyl methoxycinnamate. Not exactly
memorable names – you'll have to write them down on
your shopping list or store them in your mobile if you want
to check they are in a sunscreen before you buy it.

The best ones do both – deflect and absorb – to banish as
many rays as possible. However, no sunscreen provides 100
per cent protection, so it is good to mix in some of that
vitamin E to mop up the rays that manage to make it
through. Future sunscreens will get better at this aspect,
increasing the amount of mopping up by using antioxidants
like idebenone.

Other creams

Other than the ones I've talked about here, everything we've seen so far is just founded on pseudo-science: studies involving 30 women who are given a product and a questionnaire. That's not evidence! L'Oréal tried to use this kind of evidence to support claims their creams reduced the appearance of cellulite, and the Advertising Standards Authority threw it out. La Prairie want us to believe that putting caviar on your skin makes you look younger, without independent scientific studies to prove it, so I say you are better off eating it.

☆ *Tip*

☆ It is impossible for collagen to get in through the skin.

Jargon & ad-speak

Within the European Union, manufacturers must list all the ingredients on the packaging of a beauty product. This would be useful if people could recognize them, but companies often use the chemical names for things. So instead of seeing 'vitamin E' you see 'tocopherol acetate'. It really needs to be simplified, so that when you go into a pharmacy or department store you can make some informed decisions. I hope that this gets sorted out at some stage.

You don't want to know about extracts of caviar and jellyfish – who knows what they do? I'm open-minded about these things for the future, but I don't like the way the public gets sold misleading information. I read recently in the paper that L'Oréal had been claiming their creams reduced expression lines, but when they were asked by the advertising regulators to prove it they couldn't come up with enough evidence. So they were asked to change their ads, but what about all the people who had bought these creams already?

☆ Tip

☆ Next time you are shopping for face creams, put your sceptical hat on and use my science-speak guide to help you determine which lotions and potions are worth the money.

Science-speak devised to confuse people

Scientifically proven

Vague description designed to impress.

Data on file

The company has its own data in its own file. Unless that is
approved independently or published, it doesn't prove anything.

Published in a medical journal

Depends on what is published. Could be an advertisement!
Studies are usually reviewed by other doctors so results are
trustworthy.

Permanent (on a cream)

No such thing as a cream that can have a permanent effect.

Test done in vitro/laboratory tested

This usually means on petri dishes or animals, definitely
not on humans. It is not possible to say that positive results
obtained in the lab mean good results in humans, although
the companies would like us to think so!

Clinically proven

Vague term not to be trusted. It doesn't mean anything.

Guaranteed results

Specific term not to be trusted. Nothing in life can be guaranteed.

Cellulite disappears

Distrust any claims for cellulite or lines fading and disappearing.

Doctor-approved

Dentists can call themselves doctors, and so can anyone with a PhD, therefore this statement is meaningless.

Look for:

Double-blind crossover trial

Indicates extremely thorough testing. The results are usually reliable.

A word from this patient of mine, who has remarkably good skin . . .

I'm on damage limitation because I used sunbeds and played a lot of tennis. I'm a single mum – I had a child too young – and I work in promotions and modelling. I'm 30 now but I was 22 when I decided to start looking after my skin. I have a lot of natural fats in my diet (I've got a lot of nutrition books) and I eat lots of oily food: fish, nuts and seeds. Skin creams can't work in isolation; you've got to eat the right things too. I do sunbathe, but only with sunscreen on, and I don't sunbathe my face. I've been religious about using my creams and minimizing the time I spend in the sun.

I was on the contraceptive pill and I was getting brown marks on my face. I started reading into it and now I use the glycolic-acid lotion daily. I wouldn't miss a day – I wouldn't be so reckless! I use a glycolic cleanser – it's a higher percentage than the ones you get off the shelf. I think it has paid off. I don't think it's good to use too many products. That just over-sensitizes the skin. It's better to keep the routine simple, and stick to it.

I also go for glycolic-acid peels at the clinic – a course of six, twice a year. I find it really evens out my skin tone. I use any kind of sun protection, as long as it's high and it covers UVB and UVA. My skin tone is better and my skin feels less bumpy.

Microdermabrasion

What it is

It is a mechanical way to exfoliate your skin more deeply than you could achieve with a loofah or scrub at home, deeply enough to stimulate the production of new skin. The first one I ever saw was in Europe about 15 years ago. It was a looping tube down which crystals were blown across a little hole. Any dead skin cells and debris got sucked back up the tube – it sounds a bit primitive, but it worked. The microdermabrasion machines we use now, however, are a lot more efficient.

How it works

It is effectively a gentle, skin-friendly method of sandblasting the skin. Older technology uses aluminium or salt crystals, but the very latest machines are much easier to use, more reliable and exfoliate deeper, so they get better results: they have a small hand-piece containing industrial diamonds that pass over the skin, while a vacuum gently sucks up any debris. The skin gets a much deeper level of exfoliation than you would be able to achieve at home with a loofah or a scrub.

It is a bit like using a pumice stone to remove blemishes and smooth off rough bits of skin. By polishing off the superficial layers of skin you smooth the complexion, and if you do this repeatedly it increases the rate your skin makes new cells, which makes it look plumper and firmer.

I often use microdermabrasion as a first line of treatment. By polishing off the top skin layers we make it easier for other treatments and skin products to get further into the skin so they can be more effective.

☆ *Tip*

☆ Don't get dermabrasion and microdermabrasion muddled up. They are not the same thing. Dermabrasion refers to the now outdated and primitive technique of using a wire brush as a method of skin resurfacing. The same effect is now achieved in a more controlled way using lasers and deep peels.

Where on the body?

Skin all over, but the commonest treatments are the sun-exposed areas: the face, neck, hands and chest.

What to expect

This treatment makes the skin look healthy and more radiant immediately after you have had it done, and after six treatments any fine lines and wrinkles will be made to look less obvious because of the plumping effect. The polishing away of sun-damaged skin evens out your skin tone.

Anne

I'm 49. I have very oily skin, and sun damage that looks like lots of little dark patches, but I've seen a miracle on my face. You have to go really close to see the sun damage now. I've been having regular microdermabrasion treatments and I've changed my whole approach to tanning. It's really worked. My skin is a million times better. I started off with one session a week for the first few weeks, and now I keep the problem at bay with a treatment every month.

Microdermabrasion doesn't hurt at all; it's a pleasurable experience. You can chat to the therapist while you're having it done, and afterwards she puts on moisturizer and sun protection for you. Sometimes if I'm meeting a friend for lunch I leave my eye makeup on to save time.

It's quite a flexible treatment. They can change the heads for different parts of the face to allow for variations in the thickness of the skin, so you don't run the risk of a broken vein. At some sessions, if I feel certain areas are looking worse, I get the therapist to concentrate on those bits.

Straight after I've had it done, my skin looks clean and bright because the dead layers have come off, and it's puffed up so the little lines around my eyes look slightly thinner and softer. I have to put a high-factor sunscreen on, particularly if I'm paying golf during the following week, and I always make sure I leave it a week before going on holiday somewhere sunny. Once I was a bit naughty. I was on a bus without my sunhat and my sun damage got really bad, just from the sun coming through the window during the journey. All those treatments ruined in one day! I had to have a bit of a microdermabrasion blitz to get it back to how it was before. Six months' work can be ruined by an alfresco lunch, so you have to be careful, but my skin looks so clean and bright I think it's worth it.

When I go on holiday I wear a hat and a high-factor sun cream. I get a bit of colour but I don't bake my face in the sun any more – those days are over. I look at these ladies on the beach and the skin on their bodies looks like leather. I think a dark tan is old-fashioned now anyway, and you can get a good fake tan for a special occasion.

One thing I would say is it is not for all skin types. A friend of mine was so impressed with what it did for me she went along, but because she had highly sensitive, thin skin she was offered a red-light treatment instead. Not everyone is an ideal candidate. People need to check whether their skincare is compatible with microdermabrasion.

Microsclerotherapy

What it is

Sclerotherapy was first used in the early 1930s for treating varicose veins, but it is not used for varicose veins any more, because surgery has advanced since then and surgical removal of varicose veins gets better results. Microsclerotherapy works much better on a smaller scale, treating little thread and spider veins.

These smaller veins appear mainly on the thighs. We usually have a genetic tendency to get them and they are sparked off by a lot of standing, sitting, an operation, a past injury or a pregnancy. People get them in pregnancy because the baby weight leaning on the veins stops the blood flowing back to the heart, which makes the pressure in the leg veins build up. The same thing happens if you are overweight.

How it works

A harmless solution is injected through a micro-needle into the blood vessel. The chemical destroys the blood-vessel lining and the immune system takes away the debris.

☆ *Tips*

- ☆ If you are prone to thread veins, don't sit still on the floor for a long time with crossed legs. Keep moving. Fidgeting is a good idea.
- ☆ Don't let anyone use microsclerotherapy on your face because it can cause scarring or pigment changes. These would only be tiny but any marks made on the face are not acceptable. You can hide a mark on your legs but not on the face.

Side-effects

Bruising and blotchiness afterwards, for one to two weeks, is usually the only side effect. Very occasionally you get other little marks that take a bit longer to fade (see also the chapter on Legs for more detail).

What to expect

This works better than lasers do on thread veins. It works really well. After two to four sessions, the thread veins blanch and gradually fade. You made need top-up sessions in future to catch any new ones.

Rachel

I could see all these navy lines on my legs in the summer when I wasn't wearing tights, and I had a big group of them where I'd hurt myself falling out of a caravan when I was younger.

I was a bit wary about what the treatment would feel like, but I couldn't really feel anything. The lady said it might prick a bit but it was nothing. I could see the injection going in because it makes the skin rise, and I could feel the liquid dribbling through. I had about ten veins injected because that's about all you can have in one session.

Afterwards she put a cotton-wool pad on each one and I had to keep these on for the rest of the day. I could feel it stinging for a little while but it was OK. Then I took the pads off and put some support tights on. I wore these during the day for a fortnight and couldn't have hot water on my legs for seven days. Within a week of going to the clinic, the veins were completely gone but I had to go back six weeks later to get the rest done. I had about ten sessions in the end, one every six weeks.

My legs look fine now, and that was four or five years ago. The first time I had to go back was at the beginning of this year, because a navy vein came up on the top of my leg, but I got it sorted straight away. I think it was worth the money. Now I go around examining people's legs and thinking they should have their veins done. My tip for a friend would be: don't go in trousers because the pads are quite big, you're better off in a long skirt.

Radiofrequency Remodelling

How it works

Radiofrequency has been used for 70 years as a surgical tool for sealing blood vessels, and for a couple of years as a no-surgery treatment. Radiofrequency waves are long, so they can travel quite far into the skin, where they can heat things up without damaging the surface.

If you heat collagen to a certain temperature it does two things: contracts – reduces in length – and stirs the cells into producing more collagen. The new collagen takes between one and three months to grow, so it is during the second and third month after treatment that you can expect to notice your skin looking smoother and plumped up. However, from the moment you have the treatment loose skin gets tightened, so you will also see an immediate improvement. The long-term benefits are not yet known, but it is estimated that the effects last up to two years and quite possibly longer.

There are different systems that can deliver these radiofrequency waves, so costs, experiences and their capabilities vary. Depending on what you are treating and which radiofrequency system your practitioner is using, you'll need between three and four sessions for skin tightening on the face. It seems to take longer to have an effect on the body than on the face, which may be because the skin on the body is generally more lax, so the body will need in the region of six to eight sessions.

Some radiofrequency machines have a different hand-piece and a different power setting to makes the waves get longer, so they can get deeper into the skin and disrupt the fat cells. This aspect of radiofrequency treatment is showing very promising signs of success, but it is in the early stages of development so you will have to be patient while it is being thoroughly tested.

It is also possible that radiofrequency could be useful for reducing cellulite. Again, this hasn't been proven in independent studies yet; we only have anecdotal and photographic evidence, but I am planning to set up a study to look at benefits and side-effects.

Current data shows radiofrequency treatments don't work at all on about 10 per cent of people – and we don't know why. However, all the patients I've treated say their skin feels very different after the treatment: a softness and smoothness that seems to last.

Side-effects

Afterwards, the skin looks a bit red because you are heating it, but this only lasts for one or two hours. It is like a rosy glow. In theory, if the practitioner was really careless he could hold the pointer over the skin too long and cause the fat to disperse, which would give you a dent, or he could burn the skin, but I've never heard of this happening. Patients say the skin feels tight afterwards, but that's a bit of swelling, which settles down within a few hours.

Where on the body

- ☆ forehead lift
- ☆ around the eyes, top and bottom
- ☆ cheeks (good results)
- ☆ jowls
- ☆ neck
- ☆ anywhere on the body where there is cellulite or loose skin
- ☆ batwings
- ☆ tummy (if you are post-pregnancy or recently lost weight)

Common myth

Lifting serums

Now be honest, can you imagine a serum lifting your tummy, jowls or chest? Of course not, and any tightening on the face is probably due to moisturization and only likely to last an hour or two at the most.

Does it hurt?

It is a deep-heat sensation, but the machine I have has a cooler to make patients more comfortable. If the pointer is rolled over the skin quite quickly and kept moving it is more comfortable than if it is held still. The heat builds gradually and then has to remain at the ideal temperature in the area you are targeting for about a minute. The practitioner can determine the temperature of your skin because there is a built-in laser thermometer, and if you feel uncomfortable at any point you can just ask him to lift the pointer off.

Rachel

I am 38 years old, and I didn't expect the changes I saw in my cheeks. I had a gathering of loose skin that I noticed when I looked sideways or tipped my head forwards. I was expecting wrinkles, but suddenly I could see these jowls coming. I was at the point where I was thinking, I have to get this sorted, it is really bothering me. My mum used to say you never realize what you've got until it's gone, and I thought it was mumbo jumbo but now it's happening to me … I think it's quite scary actually.

I had the treatment six months ago and this is how long it takes to see the full results. I'm really happy with it. I think the expense is worth it because you don't have to go under the knife to get what you want. What I didn't expect was the structural improvement to the skin. I would definitely have it done again and I would even recommend it to someone who has had surgery.

When I was in the clinic I saw the girl who went in before me who'd had it on her eyes – I couldn't believe the difference. Her eyes were opened up. I was really shocked. I went in and got on the bed. The machine had a probe on the end, which the consultant moved across my face. It was quite time-consuming. He was obviously targeting the bad areas. It was a funny sensation: a wee bit of heat but nothing uncomfortable. I was quite surprised because you expect a more severe thing when the results are so extreme. I felt like he was working each little area at a time and going over and over it. I must have been lying down with my eyes closed for about an hour and a half.

My skin looked very refreshed the minute I got up: I could really see the improvement. There was an immediate lift around the lower cheek and chin area in a short space of time after the treatment. Then it was slow. I could see slight changes about a month later, and then about three and a half months later I saw quite a big change again. It is still changing slowly. Even my partner has noticed it. I'm going to have it done again in a couple of years, if it means avoiding going under the knife. Last year I was ready for that but this has definitely made a difference. I'm more than pleased.

I would recommend it. It's amazing. Even the skin seemed smoother and more glowing and that's stayed, and I find I don't have to go to have filler as often. It's one of the easiest treatments to have because it's not sore, just a bit time-consuming depending on the size of area. I would say it was preventative: use it to get your sagging under control sooner rather than later because it might not work as well if you leave it to get worse.

Sally

I'm 45 and my cheeks are sagging. They've been bothering me for about a year, but I think I'm too young to have a facelift.

When I had the treatment, sometimes it was fine because he was continually moving it over my face and I knew the heat was doing me good, so I put up with it. But there were moments when it got too hot. There were little hot spots – some bits seemed to heat up more than others. I just said, 'That's hot!', so he moved it and the heat wore off after a second or two. I looked a bit red for an hour but I went out straight after it.

I'm a beauty-feature journalist for a newspaper and a celebrity makeup artist, so I am picky and cynical, but when I woke in the morning I saw a 40 per cent improvement, and now, four days later, I'd say it was a 60 per cent improvement overall. It's amazing, to be honest. And I've been told that in another couple of months it might improve more. I would recommend it: it's like a mini facelift but without the downtime.

The Future

So that is what we have at present, but things are developing fast. Going on current research, I think the no-surgery clinic of the future will be able to offer you much more:

A more personalized service

☆ Skin products tailored to your skin by analysing it to determine its particular chemical composition.
☆ Computerized reports, based on a sample of your skin, that update you on its cell condition and the level of sun damage it has been getting – and warn you of any problems so you can take preventative action. And we'll be able to use the skin sample to pre-test for treatment effectiveness and any adverse reactions.

What I would like to see are centres that offer a one-stop shop for your health and beauty needs, where we have doctors, fitness areas, dentists, aestheticians, stylists, image consultants and surgeons, all in the one building, like a health and beauty supermarket. I expect it won't be long before there are chains like this.

Less downtime

More work is being done on new technologies that don't need a recovery time, like light and radiofrequency treatments. A new type of 'pepper-pot' laser has just come out in the US. It's designed to do the same job as a burning laser, but instead of burning off a layer it burns little holes. It takes repeated treatments to work, but this makes the recovery time amount to hours rather than weeks.

Faster treatments & quicker results

Lots of work is happening on the development of higher-speed lasers that can remove hair and rejuvenate skin much faster and with quicker results than those we have now.

More you can do at home

You can already buy blue-light lamps to treat acne at home, and it probably won't be long before there are domestic red-light versions you can treat yourself to.

More research

Scientists are working to make creams more effective without making them more irritating, by developing new formulations and increasing the level of absorption. Cosmetic companies are already becoming more 'medical' – less 'fluffy' – when it comes to developing new products and ranges. They are starting to design beauty products to be more effective on the lower layers of the skin. L'Oréal have recently bought a medical skin company so they can expand their range in this direction, and Allergan, the makers of botox, have launched this kind of skincare products in the US. Other big brands are bound to follow.

Genetic research

We have genes that determine how much pigment we have in our skin. They make our hair grey and our skin fair or dark. It is not beyond the bounds of possibility that we will at some point be able to change the gene that determines the colour of our skin – alter it to produce more protective pigment, and even take a skin sample to pop in the bank for growing our own stem cells when we need them.

Longer-lasting treatments

Botox that worked for six to twelve months would be ideal,
and hopefully a needle-less way of injecting it, using a gun
that forces air plus botox through the skin and into the
muscle – this is already used for some vaccinations. And at
some point the developers will crack the problems with
existing long-lasting fillers and produce one designed to last
around eighteen months that isn't going to give you an
allergic reaction. In addition, growing our own collagen-
producing cells may well, with a bit of refining, become a
viable long-term alternative.

Hope

The future brings hope to help treat those resistant cases of
melasma (the mask of pregnancy) and dark circles under
the eyes that we can't treat at the moment. A no-surgery
treatment for this and for the dreaded stretch mark is
already lurking on the horizon – the skin-rejuvenation laser
with a pepper-pot effect could prove to be the solution for
both problems.

Long-term removal of unwanted grey and blonde hair is
an obvious next step for IPL and laser developers, and
methods of reducing fat using ultrasound and injectables

will provide good alternative no-surgery treatments for liposuction – but don't get too excited: you will still have to diet and exercise!

There is also lots of work going on to develop no-surgery treatments for acne sufferers. These include treatments that use radiofrequency and lasers to reduce the grease-producing cells, alongside some interesting work that involves putting bacteria onto the skin – a sort of germ warfare against acne.

The trend overall is to develop techniques and treatments that are even faster, more effective and more comfortable than we have now. All good news for nervous girls!

Useful Contacts

Make sure the salon or clinic you go to is registered with the Healthcare Commission or you will have no redress if things go wrong:

National Health Regulatory Authority
www.healthcarecommission.org.uk
Tel: 0207 448 9200

To find your nearest cosmetic doctor:
British Association of Cosmetic Doctors
www.cosmeticdoctors.co.uk
Tel: 0800 328 3613

To find a surgeon:
British Association of Aesthetic Plastic Surgeons
www.baaps.org.uk
Tel: 0207 405 2234

To find a dermatologist:
British Association of Aesthetic Dermatologists
www.bad.org.uk
Tel: 0207 383 0266

To check a doctor's licence:

General Medical Council

www.gmc-uk.org

Tel: 0207 580 7642

To search 'non-surgical cosmetic procedures'
for information:

Department of Health

www.dh.gov.uk

To find cosmeceutical products:

www.skin-health.co.uk

Tel: 0870 850 6655

Court House Clinics

www.courthouseclinic.com

Index

Index